Pelican Book

10654821

SLEEP

Ian Oswald was born in Middlesex in 1929. The family
moved around the country and he received his late
school education in a 'co-ed' grammar school at Belper,
Derbyshire, where his wife was a contemporary. He
interrupted his medical training at Cambridge to study
psychology, obtaining First Class Honours, and went on
to Bristol University and various medical posts. His
research into sleep began while he was in the R.A.F.
medical branch. A Beit Memorial Research Fellowship
took him to the Institute of Experimental Psychology
at Oxford, 1957–9, since which time he has been a
member of the Department of Psychiatry, University
of Edinburgh. He is also Consultant Psychiatrist at the
Royal Infirmary of Edinburgh. In 1965–7 he worked in
Australia, establishing a Department of Psychiatry in
the Medical School at Perth.

Ian Oswald has received Doctorates from Cambridge
(M.D.) and Edinburgh (D.Sc.) Universities. He is
married and has four children.

SLEEP

Ian Oswald

PENGUIN BOOKS

Third Edition

Penguin Books Ltd, Harmondsworth,
Middlesex, England
Penguin Books Inc., 7110 Ambassador Road,
Baltimore, Maryland 21207, U.S.A.
Penguin Books Australia Ltd, Ringwood,
Victoria, Australia
Penguin Books Canada Ltd, 41 Steelcase Road West,
Markham, Ontario, Canada
Penguin Books (N.Z.) Ltd,
182–190 Wairau Road,
Auckland 10, New Zealand

First published 1966
Reprinted 1966, 1968
Second edition 1970
Reprinted 1972
Third edition 1974
Reprinted 1976
Copyright © Ian Oswald, 1966, 1970, 1974

Made and printed in Great Britain
by Hazell Watson & Viney Ltd,
Aylesbury, Bucks
Set in Monotype Plantin

Contents

Do but consider what an excellent thing sleep is:
it is so inestimable a jewel that, if a tyrant would give
his crown for an hour's slumber, it cannot be
bought: of so beautiful a shape is it, that though a man
lie with an Empress, his heart cannot be at quiet
till he leaves her embracements to be at rest with the
other: yea, so greatly indebted are we to this
kinsman of death, that we owe the better tributary,
half of our life to him: and there is good cause
why we should do so: for sleep is the golden chain
that ties health and our bodies together. Who
complains of want? of wounds? of cares? of great
men's oppressions? of captivity? whilst he
sleepeth? Beggars in their beds take as much pleasure
as kings: can we therefore surfeit on this
delicate Ambrosia?

THOMAS DEKKER
The Guls Horn-Booke, 1604

Introduction

Why do we sleep? Only at the end of this book shall I point to some answers. Sleep is imperative for mental and physical health. If deprived of it we may become mentally disordered till its restorative virtues are once more enjoyed.

Any modern physiologist can explain the function of sweating, breathing or excreting urine. Yet he knows little of the reasons why we should sleep. In this book special attention will be drawn to the methods of study that have been used to investigate sleep. Many observations will be described, but the interpretations that are drawn should always be read with a spark of scepticism, for in fifty years' time many of the interpretations may be regarded as erroneous.

What is sleep? It is a recurrent healthy state. It is a state of inertia and unresponsiveness. You do not respond overtly – having drowsed off during the sermon, you no longer fiercely nod agreement. Covert responses too are diminished – the brain no longer makes the private, inner responses which must underlie what we call perception of the outside world.

What happens when we fall asleep? The eyelids close and the pupils become very small. The secretion of saliva, of digestive juices, and urine, falls sharply. The total flow of air breathed is diminished. The heart slows. The electrical brain waves change in character, reflecting a deterioration in the efficiency with which the brain can deal with the world around. Consciousness is lost, but it is a temporary loss, for, unlike the state of anaesthesia, or coma after a severe head injury, a sufficient new stimulus – an alarm clock or a smart jab in the ribs – will cause the return of wakefulness.

Activity Rhythms

All creatures, great and small, have periods of activity and periods of inactivity. While a snail is slithering towards the lettuces, it is obviously awake. When we find it tucked snugly away within its shell beneath a boulder, is it then asleep? A question like this can lead to interminable arguments. We can really only apply the word 'sleep' with confidence to the higher vertebrates. Birds certainly sleep and many do so while standing on one leg with their head tucked beneath one wing. Most observations, however, relate to mammals, not all of which sleep like we do. Cows, for example, sleep with their eyes open and go on chewing the cud (see p. 102). We do not usually keep our eyes open, but we do keep our ears open. Dolphins have attracted a lot of research in recent years and appear to sleep for a couple of hours with first one eye, and then the other, open.

Regularly recurring inactivity in mammals is usually accompanied by sleep. Usually, but not always, for animals which hibernate in winter do not enter a state of true sleep, but a state of internally-controlled hypothermia. They let their body temperature fall to so low a level that their inner workings are all slowed down. They are fortunate enough to possess special thermostats which prevent the temperature falling to lethal depths.

The recurrence of inactivity every twenty-four hours constitutes a rhythm which the body has 'learned' through experience. We do not seem to be born with a definite twenty-four-hour rhythm. Were we born into a world where light and darkness alternated every thirty-six hours, we should probably acquire a thirty-six-hour rhythm – though such things as the urinary bladder capacity have obviously evolved to suit a twenty-four-hour rhythm. By contrast, there are other regularly recurring bodily and mental changes which certainly do not have a learned periodicity. The menstrual cycle is an example, where, about every twenty-eight days, not only do obvious physical functions alter, but mental ones too. It has been shown that women get into trouble with the police, and schoolgirls get misconduct marks, that accidents, suicide attempts, and emergency admissions to hospital, all occur more frequently in the few days just before and during menstruation than at other times of the month. There is another small peak on the statistics chart at the time of ovulation, about the middle of the month.

Even the first days of life are pervaded by rhythms of activity. Two Chicago scientists, one of whom, Dr Nathaniel Kleitman, has carried out more research into sleep than any other living person, studied the activity of babies in the first months of life. At first, an hourly periodicity revealed itself, seemingly inborn. If the baby was on demand-feeding, and not a rigid clock schedule, then he tended to demand or yell for food at some multiple of that hourly cycle. Little by little, under the pressures of social life, and the influence of light and dark, as the months passed, he spent fewer and fewer minutes moving during the night and stayed awake longer and longer by day. He had acquired, or had learned, a twenty-four-hour rhythm. Had he been, let us say, a rural Mexican baby, he would eventually have learned a rather different rhythm from a London resident: an afternoon siesta would have to become part of his normal social life.

In order to carry out learned operations, we need the grey matter of our brains, the cerebral cortex. Dogs learn twenty-four-hour rhythms of sleep and wakefulness, as we do. When Kleitman surgically deprived dogs of the cortex or outer layer of their brains, the learned rhythms were lost. After recovering fully from the actual operation, they spent much of their time asleep and woke only at irregular intervals when they paced around, deposited their excreta, ate and drank whatever was available, and then slept again. They seemed also not to dream. The twitching of the face, the growling, and the flicking of the tail, that we often see in our own dogs slumbering before the fire, were absent.

Apart from the cerebral cortex, other regions deeper within the brain are involved in acquired twenty-four-hour rhythms. If the body temperature of a healthy person is recorded each hour, it is not always the 37·0°C that the clinical thermometer indicates as the normal. During the small hours of the morning it falls to 36·0°C or below. Around midday it may rise to 37·4°C. If the amounts of chemicals in the urine, such as potassium or certain hormones, are measured every couple of hours, these too show a regular rise and fall each twenty-four hours. Suppose a man were to go on night-shift, what would happen? Provided he stayed on night-shift working long enough, his twenty-four-hour rhythms would reverse and his temperature, for example, would reach its highest point during the night. Bodily activity is more important than the alternation of light and dark in determining these rhythms, which are found in blind as well as sighted persons.

Our inner thermostats are located in the part of the brain called the hypothalamus. Here too are sensitive receptors which keep a constant check upon the concentration of chemicals in our blood and have the power to control, through the pituitary gland and its secretions into the blood, what chemicals pass from the kidneys into the urine.

A party of English physiologists went to spend a summer on the island of Spitzbergen, where daylight was continuous throughout the twenty-four hours. Half the party wore special wrist watches which were made to show the passage of twenty-four hours when, in fact, only twenty-one hours had passed. Living separately, the other half had watches that told them twenty-four hours had passed when, in reality, twenty-seven hours had gone by.

Their twenty-four-hour bodily rhythms were firmly ingrained, with the result that after a couple of days their bodily functions were six hours out of step with their untruthful watches. Their inner clocks knew better. As the days passed (if one can use that expression of Spitzbergen in summer) internal adjustments took place until the biological clocks of one party were now on a twenty-one-hour schedule and those of the other on a twenty-seven-hour schedule. But whereas the temperature control got adjusted within a week or so, in some members of the party six weeks were required to adjust the potassium excretion in the urine to the new rhythms of life. It was possible to infer that different bodily functions were not under a common control of rhythmic periodicity, that separate mechanisms in the hypothalamus must be responsible.

Of more immediate practical importance is the twenty-four-hour rhythm of alertness as it affects skill. You cannot display your abilities to best advantage except during a certain portion of the twenty-four hours. First thing in the morning and late in the evening, you are less efficient than around midday. Even if thoroughly awakened in the night, you cannot expect to perform at your peak. It may be traditional to play cards late at night, but when Kleitman set volunteers the task of rapidly sorting and dealing cards at various times of the twenty-four hours, he found that performance steadily improved as the middle of the day drew near, to decline again with the approach of evening.

If you are suddenly transferred from day-time work to night work, the ingrained rhythms of the nervous system become at once inappropriate. By day, you tend to feel wakeful and so find it difficult to rest adequately, by night you feel sleepy and cannot give of your best. Some French scientists carried out an experiment which illustrates the sort of technique which psychologists use to reveal such small impairments in skill.

Volunteers were faced with a twenty-five-minute task. Close to hand was a lever which could be pushed into any one of five positions. On to a screen the numbers 1 to 5 could be flashed in random order. In response to each number, the lever had to be moved into the appropriate position. As soon as it had reached the correct position, the next number flashed up. Instructions to be as quick and accurate as possible were given. Each individual carried out the test on four days when full nocturnal sleep was allowed. Then he had to do it again on four consecutive nights when he was allowed as much sleep as he could get during the day. The sleep by day did not prevent impairment showing itself in the small hours of the morning when, time and again, there would be a long pause, or lengthy reaction time, following the appearance of a new number. It was because the experimenters had designed a task in which no respite was allowed that it was possible to detect this impairment. Pauses, or brief breaks in performance, are characteristic of the sleepy person (see p. 54), for whom long-continued, sustained attention is impossible.

The problem of impaired efficiency for the shift-worker is also shared by those whose business demands that they fly long distances east or west. The clock times are local times, the body's inner rhythms are those of the country of origin. As long as two weeks have to pass before the temperature rhythm adjusts, and almost as long was found to be needed for adjustment in efficiency of performance in the case of eight United States residents who flew to live in Germany and the same was true when they returned home. Next time you fly the Atlantic feel even more admiration for those patient air hostesses whose internal rhythms are all at sixes and sevens and try not to think that the pilot could be even worse affected.

Experimental work of this kind should serve as a warning. Do not assume, for example, that your skill at car-driving will be perfect during the night at a time when you would normally be asleep. You may think you can defy these firmly ingrained twenty-four-hour rhythms, but you may not be the best judge, any more than a person who has consumed alcohol is the best judge of his skill. In fact, sleepiness and alcoholic intoxication have a lot in common and reinforce one another if both are present. Either can cause diplopia, or 'seeing double', together with slurring of speech. The extremely sleepy person often appears as if drunk. He will walk into walls, mumble almost incoherently, become suddenly aggressive, and lack insight into his own failings. Many people assume they are still perfectly skilful car-drivers after small amounts of alcohol, but just as the sleepy person's deficiencies will show up on a sufficiently sensitive test which requires sustained concentration, so too a Medical Research Council team showed that even the smallest quantity of alcohol will result in detectable impairment at a laboratory test resembling driving (a task which required mock-driving, just as the Link Trainer requires mock-flying).

If, therefore, you are so unwise as to take a drink before a drive, it is less potentially dangerous to do so at midday than at a late-night party. It is, however, only less potentially dangerous.

1. Methods of Studying Sleep

Suppose a pharmaceutical firm produces a new drug which it thinks will have hypnotic (i.e. sleep-promoting) properties. First, the drug will be given to animals in varying doses. If it looks promising the day will arrive when rigorous testing on humans must begin, and the smallest dose capable of inducing and maintaining sleep must be determined. A rough guide to the latter will be provided by the dose which had been found suitable for the animals, allowance being made for the difference in body weight. Then a carefully designed trial must be embarked upon. Let us call the new drug X, and suppose that it has been decided to try out the effectiveness of a 100-milligram dose, and to compare this with the effect of a standard dose of some well-tried drug, B.

Some tablets, probably sugar-coated and capable of being easily swallowed whole, must be prepared. They must all look alike and taste alike. One batch will contain the drug B, another batch will contain 100 milligrams each of X, and a further batch will contain nothing but milk-sugar. Then either volunteers or, perhaps, persons who suffer from insomnia, must be collected and the detailed design of an experiment worked out in order to discover how each kind of tablet affects their sleep. Suppose each person came and slept in a laboratory where one could measure his sleep, and suppose each came on three nights only. If then he got the milk-sugar tablet on the first night, drug B on the second night, and drug X thereafter, the results, whatever they were, would probably be meaningless. He might have slept least well on the first night, not because the sugar tablets were less effective than, say, drug X, but because he got the sugar tablet on the first night in a strange bed when he was suffering from apprehension about the whole business. He might have slept more deeply the second night because he was exhausted after too little sleep the previous night. Another complication may arise because, if a drug alters the pattern of sleep one night, on the next night, even though that drug has left the body, sleep can be affected because of a swing towards a reverse pattern. A sort of compensation (see p. 137) can arise. So that if drug X were always given the night after drug B, some spurious notions about the action of X might arise through after-effects attributable to B.

Certainly it is complicated. Even when you have got your results and there appears to be some difference between sleep after 100 mg of X and sleep after milk-sugar, you have got to carry out calculations to determine what are the chances of the differences you have observed being purely fortuitous. If your statistical calculations show that the difference might have arisen through chance alone less than once in a hundred times, then you can infer that the difference is probably a genuine one. But no matter how clever and impressive the statistical calculations, they can never compensate for poor design of the experiment itself. It is always worth taking trouble over the planning and design of an experiment. Generally it pays to make a small 'pilot' study first, the results of which are not used in the end; to gain a little practical experience of what you had planned can reveal all sorts of snags. Then one can try and eliminate the snags before starting one's more elaborate study.

An experimental method which is sometimes adopted is to use a design like that shown below, where S = milk-sugar tablets; B = well-tried drug B tablets; $X100$ = 100 mg of new drug X tablets.

| Volunteer | | Nights | |
Number	1st	2nd	3rd
1	S	B	$X100$
2	S	$X100$	B
3	B	$X100$	S
4	B	S	$X100$
5	$X100$	B	S
6	$X100$	S	B

A design of this kind would involve at least six persons, or some multiple of six. You will see, for example, that each variety of tablets would be handicapped equally by being used on the first night. Furthermore, drug *B* would follow milk-sugar just as often as sugar would follow *B*, and so on. One would hope that spurious components in the results of the study which were really attributable to the *order* of presentation of the different tablets would cancel one another out.

A trial of this kind can in fact always be executed according to a number of alternative designs or methods, each having some advantages and disadvantages. A disadvantage of the foregoing example is that probably a laboratory could not handle all six persons on the same night. It might only be possible to manage one per week. This might introduce at least one additional uncertain factor, the weather. If the first man came in the spring and the last in the summer, the summer testees might have difficulty in falling asleep because of heat and humidity, or more noisy road traffic, and this might affect the tablet order then in use more than some preceding tablet order – one could not assume that it would not. On the other hand, if one person came every week, he could at least use the same bed, whereas if all came on the same night, some beds might be softer than others. But then again the laundry might have changed its practice of starching the sheets over the months and this just might affect sleep – and so on. Perhaps no design can be perfect!

Measuring Sleep

Throughout the preceding part of this chapter, I have referred to a hypothetical investigation for comparing sleep under the influence of different factors, namely, different drugs. How should sleep be compared? One can rely simply upon a subjective estimate, by asking each individual at breakfast-time whether he thinks he slept well, slept badly, or slept indifferently. If each says he slept 'well' after one sort of tablet, and if each says he slept 'badly' after another, then clearly the pharmaceutical firm will be pleased or disappointed depending on which of the tablets was their new one. A simple study of this kind is the most necessary for many medical purposes. But if we want objective evidence about their sleep – how long they took to drop off, how long they slept, how often and when they awoke in the night, and what sort of quality of sleep it was – then we must find some criterion of the presence or absence of sleep and some method of measurement. This becomes even more important if we wish to conduct research into the fundamental nature of sleep.

One convenient measure that has often been used is provided by the number of times the individual moves in the night. Immobility is an obvious sign of sleep. A convenient method is to attach a sensitive microphone to the central bed springs. Any movement of the bed will be picked up by the microphone. A cable from it can be run to another room. The tiny electro-magnetic disturbances created can be amplified and then recorded by some form of moving pen writing on paper which is slowly, steadily and automatically moved beneath it. In the morning, the experimenter can come along and count the number of large movements or groups of movements which occurred between specified hours.

As an example of this, at Edinburgh we compared the sleep of six mentally-ill patients and six normal volunteers of the same age and sex. Between 1.30 a.m. and 5.30 a.m., the normal people moved on average forty times, whereas the patients moved on average sixty-nine times, confirming their own claim that they suffered from insomnia. Sometimes the patients were given genuine sleeping pills and sometimes dummy sleeping pills. On average the genuine sleeping pills reduced movements to only a fifth of what they were on dummy pills.

An entirely different approach requires decisions at certain fixed intervals, say every thirty minutes, about whether the person is asleep or awake. This carries the assumption that the difference between the two states is a sharp one. Obviously, a group of persons suffering from insomnia would be expected to score highly on number-of-times-awake compared with number-of-times-asleep. But how shall we decide whether a person is awake or asleep? He might just be keeping still with his eyes closed. Unless he is snoring, simple observation is not good enough. One method that has been used to provide a criterion of being awake, or, in a modified form, a criterion of the depth of sleep, is that which involves some stimulus to which the sleeper has been asked to respond.

A small pebble dropped from a height of three feet on to the centre of a gong can serve as stimulus If the individual responds to the noise, as requested earlier in the evening, by opening his eyes, then one may infer that he was either awake, or at least sleeping less deeply before the noise than if he remains undisturbed. In modern times more sophisticated techniques are available. A loudspeaker by the bed can easily provide a short musical note of fixed loudness and the experimenter can arrange an automatic device to provide the noise so that he himself can go off to bed. Instead of being there to watch the sleeper opening his eyes, the experimenter can arrange an automatic device to make a record every time a small switch is pressed by the unfortunate individual who is trying to sleep.

The study of sleep has leaped forward in the last twenty years owing to the development of a new tool. If one looks back over the history of biology one can see again and again how the really major advances followed upon the development of some new technique, some new apparatus. In the last century, the development of first-rate optical microscopes had a profound influence upon our understanding of the function as well as the structure of living organisms, including, of course, bacteria. In this century the electron microscope is making possible revolutionary advances in the study of chromosomes, those minute structures which carry the genetic blueprints of life. Equally, the development of reliable and highly sensitive electronic devices for telling us about the electrical activity of the brain has led to some quite new ideas about sleep and dreaming.

The Brain Waves

If you take a piece of wire and attach one end to one terminal of an electric battery, then lightly flick the other end of the wire across the other battery terminal, you will hear a little crackle and see a tiny spark which tell you electricity has flowed. It flowed because there was *difference of electrical potential* between the two battery terminals. This potential difference built into an ordinary torch battery is large by biological standards. It is present because of chemical interaction within the battery. Living cells contain interacting chemicals also and they too produce tiny differences of electrical potential.

The brain is composed of a countless number of individual cells. From the brain nervous messages can pass directly or indirectly to control the function of the entire body, and certain forms of variation in these nervous messages are reflected in our state of activity: whether that of wakefulness or sleep.

If an electrical connection, usually involving a little damp, salty jelly, is made between the scalp and two small silver discs, or electrodes, placed thereon at some distance from one another, tiny moment-to-moment fluctuations of electrical potential difference between the two points on the scalp can be demonstrated. These tiny fluctuations of potential difference were first discovered by Richard Caton, a man of diverse gifts and sometime Lord Mayor of Liverpool. He used rabbits and monkeys, and in 1875 presented to a meeting of the British Medical Association in Edinburgh the results of his research, including the effect upon the brain's electrical activity of a bright light shining into the rabbit's eyes. Some fifty years later, the existence of similar electrical potentials over the human brain was established by an Austrian psychiatrist, Hans Berger of Jena.

The tiny fluctuations of potential difference between the electrodes on the scalp can be recorded on paper. If you were to take again your electric battery, and if you joined it by your wire to a galvanometer, and led a wire from the other galvanometer terminal to the opposite terminal of the battery, and if you touched that terminal with the wire, took it off again, on and off, on and off, on and off, then the needle of your galvanometer would swing to and fro, to and fro, to and fro. If you arranged to run a little ink out of the tip of the needle and made it write upon paper moving steadily beneath it, then you would get a wavy ink line which would form a record of the needle's excursions. It would also form a record of the fluctuations of potential difference between the two wires as you took one on and off its battery terminal. Similarly, a wavy ink line can serve as a record of brain electrical activity. A machine called an electroencephalograph is used. It is really just a highly sensitive galvanometer, a kind of electronic voltmeter with a needle or pen for writing out the brain waves or electroencephalogram (EEG for short). Generally, several pens are used side by side, and simultaneously, to write out the electrical activity from various parts of the scalp or from elsewhere on the body at the same time.

While the eyes are closed during relaxed wakefulness, the EEG from the back of the human head reveals rhythms at about 10 ripples (or cycles) per second. This is the so-called alpha rhythm (Figure 1). It disappears if the eyes are opened, or if the individual is suddenly shouted at, or given a difficult problem to work out. It also disappears if he becomes sleepy (Figure 1). The alpha rhythm is an indication that the brain is functioning at one particular level of efficiency, alertness or 'vigilance'. When the eyes are opened or a problem undertaken, the alpha rhythm vanishes because of a shift to a higher level of alertness on the part of the brain. When the alpha rhythm is lost in drowsiness, the brain is functioning at a lower level of effectiveness. As drowsiness passes into sleep, so the EEG waves become larger and slower, so that when they are very large and slow, with waves at 1–3 cycles per second, sleep is profound. Brief bursts of faster waves are generally mixed in with these slow waves, and, unlike the alpha rhythm, are especially prominent in recordings from the front of the head. They are an important and characteristic feature of the EEG of sleep and are known as sleep 'spindles' (Figure 1).

The EEG provides both the most sensitive index we have of the presence or absence of sleep, and one measure of the kind of sleep. By its use, one can, to within a minute or two, state how many minutes a man or woman slept, so gaining a delicate tool for use, for example, in comparing one hypnotic drug with another. It is a much more sensitive tool than that provided by measuring the number of body movements. In the comparison (see p. 18) of normal volunteers and patients troubled by insomnia, between 1.30 a.m. and 5.30 a.m., the former were awake on average twenty-three minutes, the latter seventy-six minutes.

alpha rhythm — awake

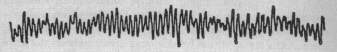

irregular little slow waves — drowsy

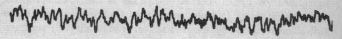

big slow waves and spindles — asleep

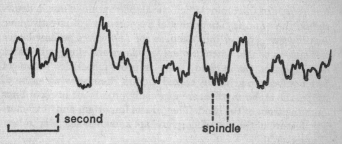

├── 1 second ──┤   spindle

Fig 1. The appearance of the electroencephalogram (EEG). The brain waves during wakefulness, drowsiness and sleep.

The difference was much more consistent among the different individuals than the difference in number-of-times-moved, and statistical calculations showed the EEG results to be significant in the sense that the likelihood of the observed difference being due to chance was less than one in a hundred.

Brain Mechanisms

The brain is encased within the skull, a hard and unyielding container. If a tumour begins to grow, if bleeding occurs, or if a part of the brain becomes inflamed and swollen because of infection, there is little room to spare. In consequence, the brain will get squashed and pushed out of shape. The space inside the skull is divided up into compartments by tough, living, tent-like flaps which are also unyielding. This means that if, because of a tumour, the brain gets squashed, it will not be squashed to a uniform extent throughout. Particular zones of the brain will get more compressed than others, according to which compartment contains the growing tumour. Obviously, if part of the brain is squashed, it cannot function properly.

It was noticed by brain surgeons that some parts of the brain, notably the cerebral cortex or grey matter, could be badly damaged without causing loss of consciousness. On the other hand, when quite small parts lower down in the brain, within the 'brain-stem' (Figure 2), were slightly squashed, the patients almost always were unconscious. Furthermore, in an epidemic illness, caused by a virus and called *encephalitis lethargica*, or sleeping sickness, which swept the world just after the First World War, the victims were overwhelmed by persistent sleepiness and tended to become wholly unrousable prior to death. Yet when the brains of those who died were examined at post-mortem, it was not the grey matter or cerebral cortex where inflammation was found. It was the brain-stem which was severely inflamed.

It seemed, therefore, that sleepiness and loss of consciousness resulted especially from impaired functioning of the brain-stem. A girl was admitted to a brain surgery hospital at Oxford in an unconscious state. Her EEG resembled that of deep sleep. It was discovered that within her upper brain-stem there was a cyst, a fluid-filled tumour. The surgeons inserted a hollow needle into the cyst and sucked out the fluid so that it collapsed (just as a grape would collapse if you sucked out its soft contents). The pressure on the surrounding normal brain tissues was thus relieved. The girl sat up and talked, apparently restored to health. Unfortunately, the fluid reformed and the cyst pressed again upon its surroundings. Again the fluid was withdrawn through a needle, again she revived, but final cure could not be achieved. The unhappy story nevertheless provides a dramatic illustration of how the welfare of a crucial part of the brain exerted a controlling influence upon consciousness. Does it mean that there is a master zone within the brain-stem for controlling sleep and consciousness?

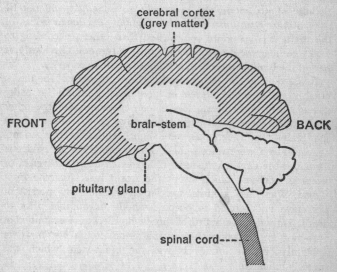

Fig 2. A diagram showing the cerebral cortex (which is actually present in the form of two large 'hemispheres', left and right) and below it the 'brain-stem', which, at its lower end, is continuous with the spinal cord. The cerebral hemispheres and brain-stem are located within the skull. The spinal cord extends down inside a bony canal within the vertebrae which make up the spinal column of the back.

While human diseases, 'nature's experiments', can teach a great deal to the doctor prepared to ponder upon the significance of what he sees in his patients, for a fuller understanding, deliberate, systematic experiments are necessary. Obviously, these cannot always be performed upon man and it is necessary to use animals.

Experiments into the brain mechanism of sleep have mainly involved cats. A Belgian physiologist, F. Bremer, in the 1930s, made a cut right through the upper brain-stem. The animal remained alive but quite inert, unreactive to smells and obviously unconscious. The pupils of the eyes were very small, as is the case during sleep, and the EEG resembled that of sleep. The brain in this condition he called the *cerveau isolé* or isolated forebrain preparation (Figure 3). In other cats, the cut across the

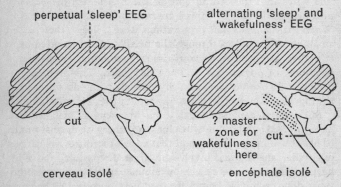

perpetual 'sleep' EEG

alternating 'sleep' and 'wakefulness' EEG

cut

? master zone for wakefulness here

cut

cerveau isolé

encéphale isolé

Fig 3. Bremer's *encéphale isolé* and *cerveau isolé*. If the connection between cerebral cortex and brain-stem was cut, EEG signs of wakefulness were never seen in the cortex. Bremer supposed this was caused by reduction of input from sense organs. Later the view prevailed that the explanation lay in a master zone for controlling sleep and wakefulness located in the brain-stem.

brain was made at its lower end, about where the spinal cord begins. This was the *encéphale isolé* (Figure 3) or whole-brain preparation. It proved very different from the *cerveau isolé*. In the *encéphale isolé*, periods of the kind of EEG normally associated with wakefulness, dilated pupils and other characteristics of what might be called 'front-end' wakefulness alternated with sleep-like periods.

What was the essential difference between these brain preparations? The fact that in one the cerebral cortex or grey matter was permanently cut off from nervous connection with the greater part of the brain-stem, wherein, we have already tentatively concluded, a master zone for the control of wakefulness and sleep could be presumed to lie. In the other preparation, the *encéphale isolé*, the cerebral cortex was not cut off from that master zone, and the alternating periods of sleep and wakefulness signs could be interpreted as attempts by that master zone to continue its customary regulation of the rhythm of life.

In the late 1940s an Italian physiologist, Giuseppe Moruzzi, was working in the U.S.A. with H. W. Magoun. They inserted fine wires into the central core of the brain-stem in *encéphale isolé* preparations. The wires were insulated except at their tips. When the *encéphale isolé* preparations were 'asleep', they passed small electrical pulses through the needle tips in an attempt to stimulate the nearby nervous tissue (a common experimental technique of physiologists). They succeeded. The preparations promptly 'woke up', the EEG rhythms changing abruptly from the big, slow waves of 'sleep' to the rapid waves of 'wakefulness'.

Subsequent experimenters, using monkeys as well as cats, have inserted similar fine wires into the otherwise normal brains of healthy animals. (I may add that such procedures are carried out under anaesthesia, involve no great discomfort, and now, having been shown to be safe by animal experiments, are sometimes done on human beings for treatment purposes.) The wires ended at terminals fixed to the scalp. A few days passed, giving time for the animals to recover fully from the operation. Then long, fine cables were attached to the terminals, leaving the animal still freely able to roam around its cage. When later the animal fell into a normal sleep, stimulating electrical pulses were passed into the brain-stem of the intact brain, just as Moruzzi and Magoun had passed them into the *encéphale isolé*. This time it was not a matter of apparent 'sleep' passing into apparent 'wakefulness' but of obvious natural sleep being superseded by very obvious natural wakefulness and activity on the part of the intact animal. Stimulating the central core of the brain-stem caused a transition from sleep to wakefulness.

Instead of stimulating the brain electrically through needles inserted into it, the experimenters could just as readily have caused awakening by more natural stimulants, such as a shout or a tug on the tail. Such procedures would have stimulated sense organs. Sense organs are known to pass information to the brain in the form of small electrical impulses passing along from the periphery. Could it be that those impulses travel to the central core of the brain-stem and by an action at that site provoke awakening?

It was known that, via relays, the impulses actually went to the cerebral cortex. Might they go to both destinations? The answer could not be found through the sort of philosophical speculation beloved by our forefathers: only systematic experiment could reveal the truth. The study of 'evoked potentials' provided the answer.

We have already seen how an electroencephalograph machine can pick up and amplify tiny electrical potentials from nervous tissue. A cathode ray oscillograph can do the same. If electrodes connected to either machine are placed upon a nerve travelling up the leg, and if then a sudden stimulus such as a bang on the big toe is given, a moment later there is a sudden, brief potential change at the recording point higher up the body. It is the 'evoked potential'. With further electrodes recording the activity of the cerebral cortex, an 'evoked potential' is found at the cortex too, a fraction of a second after it was present in the nerve lower down the body (Figure 4). Nerve messages travel fast. In practice, the big toe would get bruised, so that small, sharp electric shocks either to the skin or directly to the sensory nerve are generally used in both human and animal studies. On the other hand, the special sense organs can be stimulated in ways appropriate to them – a flash of bright light before the eyes, a loud click near the ear. Evoked potentials always follow in the nerves and brain.

Fine wires were therefore inserted into the central core of the brain-stem, into the *reticular formation*, as it is called on account of its appearance under a microscope. They were not for stimulating, but for recording evoked potentials. Others were inserted through the skull on to various zones of the cerebral cortex. An electric shock to the foot was followed by an evoked response in the cortex and in the brain-stem reticular formation. A loud click evoked responses in the part of the cortex which is specially concerned with hearing and in the reticular formation. A bright flash of light was followed by an evoked potential in the rear part of the brain, which subserves especially visual function, and,

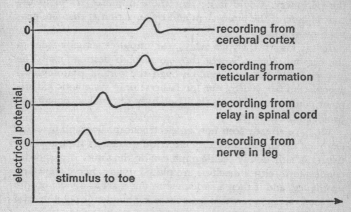

Fig 4. The electrical 'evoked potential' recorded at different points on its upward path to the brain. Notice that the nerve message from the peripheral sense organs reaches both cortex and reticular formation.

once more, in the reticular formation. So it gradually became established that all the main sensory paths from sense organs give off branches or 'collateral afferents' which turn off into the reticular formation while the main path continues, via relays, to the cortex. Once the impulses arrive in the reticular formation they probably lose any characteristics which distinguish their origin, they are all equally grist to the mill, fuel for the fires which keep the reticular formation excited. A flash of light and a shock to the foot applied at the same time do not give an extra large evoked potential in the reticular formation: the pair are submerged into a single potential which does not differ from that which would have been produced by either alone.

So here is a working hypothesis. All sense organs, when stimulated, send impulses to the brain, and always impulses branch off to excite the reticular formation, the master zone for the control of wakefulness, so that the sleeping animal becomes an awake animal. But how to confirm this? After all, the impulses go on to the cortex, could it not be these that cause awakening?

This question was answered by a group of research workers in Los Angeles. They took two groups of cats, anaesthetized them, and operated on their brains – it sounds easy, put like that, but actually involves great skill and patience. In one group, let us call it group *A*, they destroyed the upper reticular formation, taking great care not to damage the main sensory pathways from sense organs to cerebral cortex. In the other group, group *B*, they left the reticular formation intact but cut the main sensory pathways to the cortex *after* the collateral afferents to the reticular formation had branched off. The anaesthetic soon wore off and, as the days passed, there was revealed a striking difference between the two groups of cats. Group *A* cats lay in perpetual sleep, with the usual sleep EEG; the sense organs still sent impulses to the cortex, but, without the benefit of a functioning reticular formation, the cats remained in oblivion. Group *B* cats, with the reticular formation intact and open to excitement via the collateral afferents, slept from time to time. A noise would awaken them; at other times they wakened spontaneously and roamed around, obviously fully awake even though a little unsure of the world.

The essential conclusions that have arisen out of all this work by men of diverse countries, are depicted in Figure 5. All the great sensory paths to the brain give off collateral afferents to the reticular formation, along which impulses pass to help keep the reticular formation in a state of, as it were, effervescent excitement in which it gives off 'non-specific' impulses – invigorating or vitalizing impulses – which pass not only upwards to the cortex but also downwards to the spinal cord. The cortex and the spinal cord are thereby pepped up, are more able to respond efficiently – incoming information can be competently dealt with, so leading to perception and appropriate action. The muscles of the body are toned up, the mind is eagerly receptive.

The reticular formation is conceived of as a zone of nervous tissue, the excitement of which periodically undergoes both

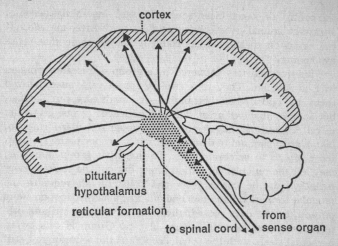

Fig 5. A diagram which represents the reticular formation being excited by impulses from sense organs via branches or 'collaterals' from the main traditional pathways to the brain. The excited reticular formation gives off streams of non-specific impulses which, for example, ascend to the cortex to increase its efficiency.

abrupt and gradual variations. In consequence, the upflow of non-specific impulses, which keep the grey matter pepped up, undergoes continual variation in intensity. It is the presence of an efficiently working cortex which makes possible 'clever' activity, learned activity, the weighing of past with present evidence, and a rational decision to embark upon, and the power to execute, skilled behaviour. Without the upflow from the reticular formation the cortex cannot serve these purposes. The intensity of the upflow can vary from very high levels, through moderate, to very low levels. A person can be in a state of efficient wide-awakeness, a state of inefficient drowsiness, or a slumbering state of total ineffectiveness. In the first, he may be capable of witty repartee, in the second of some mumbled indication of his latent powers, in the third of only oblivious snoring.

It soon became realized that quite a number of things help to keep the reticular formation excited. Whenever a sense organ is stimulated, nerve messages pass from it to the brain, some of them going to the reticular formation. If the stimulus is a particularly violent one, the reticular formation suddenly becomes very excited, and we may feel ourselves abruptly alerted. However, it does not need a loud bang to alert us, a quiet whisper can do so just as easily if the words are, for example, abusive, or in some other way specially significant for us, because the sense organs pass the messages also direct to the cortex where their significance can be assessed. The cortex can then send its own signals to the reticular formation to help excite the latter which, in turn, will then enable the cortex to deal competently with the *sequelae* to the whisper. Equally, most of us are aware how worry can keep us from sleep – the cortex sending signals to the reticular formation, so keeping the latter active – or so one would suppose.

Can we prove the existence of this route – sense-organ to cortex, to reticular formation, and then up again? We cannot trace it in its entirety by any direct method. In monkeys, it has been shown that when parts of the cortex are suddenly and artificially stimulated by electric pulses during sleep, the animal will awaken, and one may infer that messages had been passed down to excite the reticular formation.

Using Oxford students a few years ago, we tried to investigate this role of the cortex, to discover whether it could cause awakening by sending messages down to excite the reticular formation in response, not to a loud bang, but to a specially significant word. A word is a natural stimulus, unlike the artificial electrical pulses applied directly to the cortex of the monkey. How to be sure that the cortex was involved in the circuit? By ensuring that the brain had to carry out complex discriminations between different words. We know from cases of injury or disease of the brain in humans and animals that unless a certain area of the cortex is working, one complex pattern of noise cannot be discriminated from another; more particularly, speech sounds cannot be understood or responded to. So, if the brain was discriminating between words, the cortex must be doing the job.

What sort of techniques must be employed in such experiments? First, it is essential that if a person wakens from sleep the possibility that he may have done so spontaneously, and not as a consequence of your stimulus, must be borne in mind. One must therefore compare how often he appears to awaken after the deliberate stimulus, with how often he appears to waken spontaneously at comparable periods of the night. Secondly, one must bear in mind that novelty is a very potent awakener. People who have slept through continuous loud noise will often awaken if the noise stops – the silence is so different from what they have become accustomed to. Sudden awakening after calling out the sleeper's name, or even the tape-recorded voice of her child calling, *Mummy*, would not necessarily indicate responsiveness to speech. It might simply be that the quality of the noise was novel, quite different from the sounds of the preceding couple of hours (passing traffic, the sighing of the wind, the rattling of the door). The experimental stimulus must be no more novel than other noises which precede it.

We therefore made a very long tape-recording in which fifty-six names were called out one after another, over and over again in different orders, with several seconds between each name. Having persuaded a volunteer to come and sleep in the laboratory we would attach electrodes to his scalp and to his hands. He was told that if during sleep his own name, say, *Peter*, was called out, he should respond to it by clenching his hand, and that he should do the same if one other particular name, say, *David*, was called. He then fell asleep while the tape-recording was played, drowsing off through an endless barrage of words, occasionally clenching his hand as one of the crucial names came. Eventually, he fell asleep and, sure enough, would very often suddenly rouse from sound sleep and clench his fist just after either of the crucial words.

Next we had to get a man called David to volunteer. He too was asked to pick out, during his sleep, the names *David* and *Peter* from all the others (the degree of novelty of either word being no greater than that of other names adjacent in time). And so on with name-paired volunteers.

It was necessary to use pairs of people like this for they

served as 'controls' for each other, balanced each other out. It might have been that we could have recorded *Pèter* more loudly than *David*, so that had we used only Peter, he might have picked out his own name in sleep more often than *David* just because it was louder. Or because it contained more disturbing, high-pitched sounds. If, on the other hand, Peter responded much more often to *Peter* than to *David* and David responded much more often to *David* than to *Peter*, it would seem that the reason for the name being picked out in sleep was that it was David's or Peter's own name.

The upshot of all this was that, whereas spontaneous awakenings and movements (which we counted during the period of each ten names that preceded each crucial one) were very rare, fist-clenching after 'own' name had been called was so frequent that the difference could not reasonably be attributed to chance. The same was true of the 'other' name – Peter responded best to *Peter* but was also able, though with less certitude, to pick out *David* during sleep. Furthermore, even if fist-clenching did not occur, the EEG of sound sleep, with slow waves and sleep spindles, was much more often disturbed by a person's own name than by any other name. The electrical response (called a K-complex) was an indication of a sudden increase in the upflow of exciting impulses from the reticular formation to the cortex. In some additional experiments, these electrical responses in the EEG occurred much more often after any meaningful name, such as a name played forwards by the tape recorder, than after the same name made meaningless by being played backwards.

Even in the sleeping brain, the cortex evidently was getting enough help from the reticular formation to enable it to maintain a sort of unconscious scrutiny of outside noises, for it was discriminating between the names. Only the cortex would be capable of that complex task. After certain discriminations had evidently been made, selective arousal occurred. Therefore, after discrimination by the cortex, messages must have left the cortex ('Hey, this is important, you'd better help me wake up!'), travelled down to and excited the reticular formation, and then led to an increase of the invigorating upflow from it.

Incidentally, some other names during sleep were specially

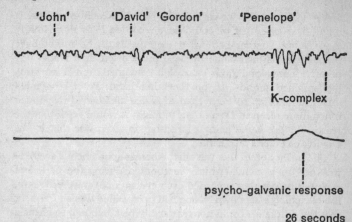

Fig 6. At irregular intervals of four to eight seconds a voice speaks names from an endless list. Big slow waves and spindles were visible in the EEG. The names *John!, David!, Gordon!* have little effect on the EEG and provoke no psycho-galvanic responses. The name of his beloved, *Penelope!*, provoked a group of big waves forming a 'K-complex' in the EEG and a surge of electric potential at the palm.

potent in leading to arousal, none more so than the name of a recent girl-friend (Figure 6). While Neville slept, the name of his recently acquired heart-throb, *Penelope*, would cause a most violent perturbation in his EEG, and a huge 'psycho-galvanic response', or sudden sweating of the palm (itching too, perhaps!).

Many other sources of reticular formation excitement have been discovered, especially chemical ones, such as excess of carbon dioxide in the blood, or a shortage of oxygen. Any interference with breathing will quickly cause awakening. Nevertheless, as we have earlier said, sleep is a condition of inertia and unresponsiveness. That unresponsiveness extends to the normal body reflexes, and the concentration of carbon dioxide in the blood that will be tolerated during sleep, without causing reflexly increased breathing, is much greater than during wakefulness. In natural deep sleep, the concentration rises higher than it does after a large dose of morphia during wakefulness, morphia being a powerful suppressant of breathing reflexes. Adrenalin, too, was found to excite the reticular formation, an illustration of a potential vicious circle, for adrenalin is a chemical released into the blood by the adrenal glands whenever the person is excited or fearful. By an action on the reticular formation it would arouse him even more, and lead to more adrenalin release by impulses passing down from the reticular formation to the spinal cord and the centres in it which control adrenalin release.

If such a vicious circle were to continue unabated, you might expect the poor chap to blow up! Fortunately, regulating devices are present which prevent the development of vicious circles. These 'homeostatic' devices illustrate a common principle, not merely within the nervous system, but throughout the whole of the bodily economy. If some mechanism, through its activity, changes a particular function in a specific direction, the mere occurrence of that change will start up other mechanisms which tend to reverse the direction of change toward the original level of function.

When adrenalin is released into the blood-stream it brings about a rise of blood pressure in the arteries (the blood vessels carrying blood away from the heart). The increased pressure causes a slight stretching of the wall in certain parts of the arterial system, notably the carotid sinus in the neck. Within the walls of the carotid sinus are organs highly sensitive to stretching. When the blood pressure rises these organs send a powerful stream of nerve impulses to the brain-stem which damp down the excited reticular formation. In this way the vicious circle referred to above would be prevented.

There are rare people who, if they twist their necks to left or right while wearing a tight collar, will become unconscious – they fall abruptly asleep because of the distortion of the carotid sinus wall! A subtler but more common sleep-promoting action of the carotid sinus may underlie a relation between atmospheric pressure and the tendency to take a nap. When you inflate a balloon its walls are stretched by a pressure from within, just as is always and quite normally the case with the arteries. If the balloon were placed in a room in which the air pressure was reduced towards a vacuum, the balloon would rapidly expand and soon explode. In the same way, if the atmospheric pressure fell slightly one could expect a very slight expansion of the arteries, particularly the carotid sinus, and therefore a tendency for sleep to be caused. Ordinarily there are a host of factors which act to keep us awake, so that any very mild sleep-promoting influences would be swamped. But what of a gentle rest period? Would resting people fall asleep more easily on low-pressure days?

Airline crew who had routine EEG tests as part of a health check-up were studied in Paris. Keeping still during such a test is a boring but restful occupation. Occasionally people will fall asleep during it, and when, in Paris, the dates upon which airmen fell asleep were checked against the atmospheric pressure, sure enough it was the days on which the barometer was low that sleep usually overcame them.

Homeostatic or regulatory mechanisms are so common in the nervous system that it is not surprising that other means have been discovered whereby the excitement of the reticular formation is damped down. Most important is the degree of pep which the reticular formation itself imparts to the cortex. The more the cortex is pepped up or 'activated', the more strongly it sends down special nerve impulses to damp down the reticular formation. Some beautifully designed experiments in Paris showed that there was no one particular part of the cortex responsible for this. The whole cortex functioned in this way, for when various areas of cortex were prevented from doing so by local, rapid cooling, the damping effect was reduced in accordance with the extent and not the site of the cooling. One would suppose that the cells in the cortex which send down these damping influences to the reticular formation are different from those which can send down exciting impulses (see p. 31), though probably if one increases the other decreases.

Consciousness

To attempt to define consciousness would be to risk the displeasure of philosophers. I am no philosopher. However, most of us know what we mean when we say we are conscious of, or aware of, something whether outside or within ourselves. It will have become apparent from all that has already been written in this chapter, that it is now believed that when human consciousness is lost it is because of failure on the part of the reticular formation to send up a sufficiency of the non-specific or 'activating' nerve impulses to the cortex.

The failure may be for entirely healthy reasons, as in natural sleep, which is a state of unconsciousness from which we can fairly easily be roused. Or it may result from abnormal causes such as pressure upon, or inflammation within, the reticular formation, the state of unconsciousness being one from which the victim cannot be fully roused. It is not strictly correct to call sleep a state of unconsciousness, for at least during some of our sleep we are conscious – not in its full sense, not of the outside world, but of an inner, or dream-world, as we shall be discussing later in this book.

The attributes of consciousness – skilled response, the utilization of former experience, a subsequent statement of having been aware, and being now able to describe what passed – these are not possible without the cerebral cortex or grey matter. Wakefulness, by contrast, is possible without a cortex. Consciousness and wakefulness are not synonymous. Animals from which the cortex has been removed (p. 11) show alternating periods of sleep and activity. While active they move about, eat and excrete and must be considered awake. There are no grounds for inferring the possession of consciousness on their part. The same is true of those human monsters which from birth lack a cerebral cortex. A few of these live, and, if cared for, survive for years, but when awake never reveal any attributes of consciousness – they merely swallow, grunt, and move their limbs aimlessly.

The most common state of human unconsciousness, during life anyway, apart from sleep is that induced by chemical anaesthetics – chloroform and ether are well-known examples. Most adults today who have general anaesthetics are 'put out' initially and very quickly by an injection into the blood-stream of a barbiturate drug like thiopentone. The drug is quickly carried to the brain by the blood. Using the evoked potential technique new light has been thrown on the action of anaesthetics. Evoked potentials were recorded from both the cortex and the reticular formation while the animals were awake. Then some were put to sleep with ether, others with thiopentone. If a stimulus, such as an electric shock, was now applied to the leg, the evoked potential in the cortex was still present without reduction. On the other hand the evoked potential in the reticular formation of the anaesthetized animals was now very small. Although the cortex still responded to the nerve impulses from the leg, the reticular formation was unresponsive. The anaesthetic drug was showing a predilection for impairing reticular formation function.

When therefore the surgeon sticks a knife into you while you are anaesthetized, your reticular formation is not merely just ticking over quietly, as in sleep, it is also slightly poisoned so that it cannot respond and cause you to awaken. However, we have already seen that numbers of different factors affect the reticular formation, not only anaesthetics: for example, chemicals like adrenalin, and exciting impulses coming down from the cortex. When I was first taught about anaesthetics as a medical student, the role of the reticular formation was not understood and I remember that as we sat in the ante-room to the surgical theatre the anaesthetist told me how puzzling it was that, if one had two people of similar size, and brought about a similar concentration of anaesthetic in the blood of each, if one patient was calm he would be the first to become unconscious. If the other was very apprehensive he would need a much bigger dose of anaesthetic. We can now realize that in the second patient, while the anaesthetic agent was trying to damp down the reticular formation, it was all the time being counteracted by adrenalin and by nerve impulses from the cortex which were trying to excite the reticular formation.

Hitherto in this chapter I have written of the reticular formation as if it were a single localized zone in the brain-stem. It is not. It is neither sharply defined anatomically, nor is it uniform in its structure and function. Later research has increasingly shown differences of function between different parts of the reticular formation. An elegantly designed experiment by Italian research workers provided a first example. The connections between different arteries to the brain were tied off before they reached the *encéphale isolé* preparation. Then the anaesthetic, thiopentone, discussed above, was injected into the arteries going to the upper brain-stem. The 'waking' *encéphale isolé* passed quickly into the 'sleeping' state. Nothing surprising about that. But if, instead, thiopentone was injected into arteries supplying only the lower brain-stem of already 'sleeping' *encéphale isolé* cats, the EEG quickly changed to a 'waking' one. Just the opposite effect. The most reasonable explanation was that the reticular formation in the lower brain-stem normally has the special function of damping down the upper part (which is the part from which impulses flow up to the cortex to make the EEG of the latter look 'awake' or 'asleep'). Knock out that damping action, by partly poisoning the nerve cells with thiopentone, and the upper reticular formation is allowed to function in a more lively manner. The demonstration of a zone which looked as if it might constantly be nudging the brain towards sleep revived interest in older work by an eminent Swiss scientist, W. R. Hess, who had electrically stimulated the thalamus, which is part of the upper brain-stem, and found that a cat would thereupon peacefully groom itself, curl up and settle to sleep. It had been an observation inconvenient to reconcile with the idea of sleep as a negative state brought about by lack of reticular formation excitement. Indeed it was tempting to brush aside what Hess had seen and attribute it solely to the strength of the electrical current used, which far exceeded any naturally-occurring brain electrical process – as is usual in this kind of work.

However, a Mexican experimenter found that sleep could be made to appear by chemical stimulation of many areas of the upper and lower brain-stem. Finally, in Los Angeles, the presence of definite sleep-promoting zones in the brain has been confirmed in a reverse manner by making tiny areas of destruction in the lower part of the cerebral hemispheres themselves. When this had been done on both sides of the brain some cats did not thereafter sleep at all and eventually died of exhaustion, while others suffered severe insomnia from which they recovered only after 6–8 weeks.

It is evident that there are a host of different mechanisms, some making for wakefulness and some for sleep (and some, as we shall later see, for two kinds of sleep). They should not be thought of as acting in opposition, as might appear from laboratory experiments. We should rather try and understand each as playing its harmonious role within a wondrous orchestra.

2. Mental Function and Sleep

In the previous chapter we reached the conclusion that the degree of excitement of the reticular formation was subject to many influences – some exciting, some damping. Many of these influences, for instance those which reflect ingrained twenty-four-hour rhythms, are as obscure as the damping influence that must be presumed to underlie the intense sleepiness which results from prolonged sleep loss. One can only suspect that some changing chemical balance may underlie these, and that chemical receptors send nerve impulses to excite or dampen the reticular formation.

In any case, it is obvious that the level of reticular formation excitement can vary from one extreme to another. There are no sharp dividing lines between being awake and asleep, being very excited, calmly reflective, pleasantly relaxed, peacefully drowsy and sweetly sleeping. These states are accompanied by variations in the level of what we call cortical *vigilance*, from high to low.

When cortical vigilance is high we are efficient. But there is an optimum high level, for if the level is too high we perform at less than peak efficiency. Hectic haste must bow to unhurried skill. When vigilance falls below the optimum we again become inefficient. There is a disorder known as narcolepsy in which the sufferer is assailed by periods of uncontrollable drowsiness during the day. When very sleepy he is inefficient. Speech may become mumbled, he cannot coordinate his gaze (he 'sees double'), he stumbles into the kerb and bumps into passers-by, much to his subsequent embarrassment.

If one gets a person to make rhythmic movements with his hands and simultaneously records his EEG, his arm muscle activity, and the extent of movement at a time when he is becoming drowsy, one sees that precisely executed and accurately timed movements accompany alpha rhythm in the EEG, but that as vigilance falls and the alpha rhythm is replaced by little slow waves his movements become weak, clumsy and disorganized. One can actually see this as a written record. What cannot be so easily depicted is the disorganization of thinking that also accompanies a fall of vigilance. Tests for this can be devised (see p. 55), but often one must rely upon descriptions immediately following a brief period of drowsiness. The individual will tell us that his attention wandered. Ideas and images (including 'mental pictures') out of context with his immediate surroundings, and inconsequential trains of association occupied his flaccid mind. Within a few moments of waking the fleeting memories of these may have vanished, for the power to store up memories depends upon the level of vigilance.

If you wish you can purchase machines for, so it is claimed, sleep-training. To learn while asleep! The student, weary of his books, his mind resting by day, absorbing by night! In essence these machines are just tape-recorders which emit spoken instruction automatically during the night. Do they work? No.

You cannot learn while asleep. Just before settling to sleep one can learn, and may learn specially effectively then, provided there is only a very limited amount to learn. Provided the sleep is not too immediate, the rest which the mind gets seems to help remembering, for consecutive mental activity interferes with memorization. If, at any time, you read one page, then another, you will subsequently be able to remember less of the first page than if, instead of having also read the second page, you had telephoned your girl-friend. Reading the second page interfered with storing up a memory of the first. If you read a page before bed, since you cannot read while asleep, you remember the page well in the morning.

But while asleep you do not learn. While drowsy you learn very poorly. The lower your cortical vigilance the worse you do. Two psychologists in the U.S.A. made a thorough test of the commercial sleep-learning claims. They played tape-recorded answers to questions during the night, always recording their volunteers' EEG. In the morning, answers which had been played while alpha rhythm was present were recalled easily.

Answers played while the alpha rhythm was waning were often not recallable. Answers played when sleep slow waves and spindles occupied the EEG could never be recalled.

Supposing the information played during sleep were repeated over and over again, would that help later recall? To test this, they drew up a list of words and, taking great care to turn off the sound whenever the sleepers' EEG showed momentary signs of raised vigilance, played the list of words again and again through the night. In the morning the volunteers were always asked if they could remember the words, but they never could. They were then given a sheet of paper with a longer list of words upon it. Mixed up in this longer list were the words played by night. 'Just pick out any words that look somehow familiar.' They tried, but those they picked out were no more often words which had been played during their sleep than the other words of the new list. Not even a vague memory persisted of that which they had had the opportunity of learning while asleep.

The lack of durability of the memories of sleep experiences prompts certain questions. Might people who say they never experience dreams at night really be people who simply forget their dreams? In Chapter 4 we shall see that this is true. Might we all spend the entire night, or most of it, with some sort of mental life in progress and then forget it? This too, as we shall see, may be the case. Then again, some people describe strange experiences while drowsy – visions, voices, bodily jerks and bizarre sensations. Do other people not have these or do we all have them, but mostly forget? I believe the latter is true. Unless one is roused, or determines to rouse oneself sufficiently to make a written record upon spontaneously stirring, all trace of these experiences is forever lost.

Hypnagogic Experiences

As slumber steals over us, our cortical vigilance does not fall at a uniform rate. It shifts up and down, tending only gradually to sag lower and lower. Alpha rhythm appears in bursts, but less and less often, with longer and longer periods of slow waves in the EEG. Little by little the control of our ideas escapes us. At intervals we 'come to', realizing we have just had some rather queer thoughts about something which was not closely related to the inner musings of a minute ago. Suddenly we may realize that we have been talking inwardly to ourselves and that we have just fathered a nonsense-phrase, perhaps containing new words (neologisms).

I once surfaced having inwardly spoken the phrase, 'Or squawns of medication allow me to ungather'. The word which here I spell 'squawns' is a neologism, as is 'ungather'. On another occasion, 'And yet it's rather indoctrinecal'. The last word is another neologism. Had I not at once written these down they would have been lost for ever. Many people are able to recount similar experiences and an amusing collection was printed in the *New Statesman* during 1960, the choicest being in, as is sometimes the case, doggerel verse. It was communicated by a Mr Singleton of London:

> 'Only God and Henry Ford
> Have no umbilical cord.'

In these instances it seemed to be the individual's own voice speaking the words. Often, however, it is someone else's voice which is experienced. An example that most people will recall is of seeming to hear one's own name called. Awakening occurs, and then it is soon realized that it was only imagination. More complex creations are customary, however. Examples given me by one young lady include:

'Those who take sideward epidemics.'
'Well, he was a dog's inn.'
'There has been something keenly interesting to that sort of spaxel.'

The voice may accompany an equally striking display of visual imagination. Many people have recorded these visions of half-sleep. Faces are common, sometimes coloured, changing and moving, sometimes seeming to pass across the field of vision. Children often are frightened by such faces in the dark. Abstract forms, cubes and patterns, nature scenes, seascapes, the varieties are endless. Especially common are those which reflect the activities of the day. After a long day's driving, there comes an endless vision of passing road, with cars and lorries.

As sleep draws nearer, the visions and voices become more complex, and many people, when roused, will describe little adventures in which they seemed to be participating, little dreams in fact, which contrast with a more spectator-like quality of the earlier moments of drowsiness.

On occasion the experiences may be brought to an abrupt end. Once I was having a vision of a red sports car backing on to a road, while inwardly saying (as I afterwards wrote down) within myself the nonsense sentence, 'Maintenance therapy was apparently backed into the road'. At the word 'road' I had a violent bodily jerk and awoke.

The sudden bodily jerk of the whole or a part of the body upon falling asleep is familiar to everyone. Usually it is forgotten. The more vivid ones are accompanied by a sudden and equally violent sensation, such as a flash of light, a loud bang, a musical note, a surge of indescribable feeling passing through the body, or a feeling of falling. The fall may seem to end with a sudden impact, or as a violent clutching for support, as if to arrest the fall – in either case there is a jerk which leaves the individual wide awake with heart pounding, a quickening of the breath and a slight cold sweat. Always it occurs when the alpha rhythm has been absent for a few seconds and small slow waves have been present in the EEG. Sigmund Freud, who regarded all dream experiences as wish-fulfilling (in my view he was wrong), proposed that, in the case of women, the falling experience indicated a wish to be a fallen woman. His explanations became tortuous in the case of men.

When a wife or husband is asked if his or her spouse has these jerks, they will nearly always report that they are much more frequent than the other realized. Most are forgotten. Some people will say that they always 'fall' with their jerks, and always as part of the same little dream – a fall down the stairs or off a wall.

Drowsiness is as often present after first waking in the morning as it is last thing at night, so all these freakish experiences are common then too. One's contact with reality has been severed for a longer period, and in the morning it may take longer to orient oneself afresh to the world of real events – one needs to pinch oneself, as it were. The visions sometimes do not at once vanish when the eyes are opened and not for a few moments is their true nature realized. Students have described how, for example, a spider was seen upon the bed, or a friend, ghost or angel standing there, only to vanish when spoken to.

Having already glimpsed the kind and degree of impairment of mental life with the oncoming of sleep, we shall return later in this book to consider how this impairment is manifest after sleep loss and during prolonged dreams.

Monotony

It has already been emphasized that novelty can cause awakening. Conversely, lack of novelty, or monotony, tends to provoke sleep. The Russian experimenter, Pavlov, in his studies of conditioned reflexes, kept dogs in a stand for long periods with conditioned stimuli being given over and over again. They kept falling asleep. 'The experimental sleep,' he wrote 'can be reproduced with the same exactitude as the reaction of a hungry dog to a piece of meat.' The sleep response is always greater if movement is restrained, whether by a harness, EEG recording wires to the head or social obligations to remain still. Few are they who can survive a boring sermon, or lecture, without suddenly realizing that they have become drowsy and that their minds have wandered.

An instructive experiment was conducted in Sweden. Thirty volunteers came twice to the laboratory and reclined in a comfortable chair for half an hour each time. They were told that their bodily functions were going to be studied during quiet and during noise. Half had the quiet time on their first visit and half on their second visit. In the noise session there were repeated loud, high-pitched bleeps, each lasting 4 seconds, and recurring about every 30 seconds. During this session of monotonously recurring signals many more subjects fell asleep, they did so more quickly and they slept longer. The minute by minute graph of sleep rose higher and higher, and always it was steeper with the monotonously recurring loud noise: statistical calculations showed that chance alone could not be held responsible for the difference. If, in fact, something is present which is of a monotonous character, but which is at least potentially of interest to you, you are more likely to fall asleep than under conditions of meaningless uniformity.

This has important implications, for there are many monotonous practical tasks, whether long-distance driving, or sitting and watching a radar screen for recurring signals, some few of which might be important, which impose restraint of movement upon the observer. Sleep is a definite hazard for truck drivers on long journeys, especially if they have been kept short of night-time sleep. As with any biological function there are big individual differences. Some people drowse off more easily than others. In Czechoslovakia it was discovered that two-fifths of a sample of long-distance truck drivers were known to have had at least one near-accident owing to falling asleep. These men described hypnagogic hallucinations while driving, described a greater need for sleep than their fellows and, when given complex mental tasks in their off-duty hours, they performed less well than other drivers.

Arduous and more or less endlessly repeated tasks make heavy demands on anyone. During the Berlin air-lift, the constant ferrying under conditions of anxiety, and with only make-shift facilities for the aircrew, who found themselves unable to get a sufficiency of sleep in quiet surroundings, led to such signs of strain that a special investigation into aircrew fatigue was carried out, with consequent improvements in their working conditions, and sleeping quarters, improvements which helped to ensure the successful maintenance of the operation.

The soothing action of repetitive or rhythmic stimulation can be seen in many guises. The old lady in her rocking chair. The baby rocked in its mother's arms. Even rhythmic gum-chewing has been shown by experimental psychologists to cause relaxation. Rhythmic rocking as an avenue of escape from harsh reality to slumbrous tranquillity occurs spontaneously in young primates. Young chimpanzees or monkeys, taken from their mothers and put into a strange and frightening room, crouch down on their haunches and rock rhythmically to and fro. Just as some human infants who feel lonely when put to bed will comfort themselves by sucking their thumbs, others (who less often suck their thumbs) rock themselves to sleep. This is quite common in 6–18-month-old infants and you may have known an infant who would either roll rhythmically from side to side, or who, resting on hands and knees, would bang his head rhythmically on to the pillow or cot-head. In the latter case so much noise may be made that the whole household, and the neighbours, are disturbed. Often the children make crooning noises at the same rhythm. Generally they cease to do it as they grow older, only occasionally continuing into later life, when the rocking may take place, not only before, but actually *during* sleep. In 1880 a Dr Putnam-Jacobi in New York described a boy of three and a half who rocked rhythmically in his sleep for hours. Yet in the morning 'the child would seem in nowise fatigued . . . the rotations only took place during a very sound sleep'. Even adults do it sometimes (p. 69).

Provided new decisions are not required, simple rhythmic movement can continue during sleep. Cows, sheep and other ruminants go on ruminating, or rhythmically cud-chewing, while asleep. There are many stories of soldiers marching in their sleep and in a famous nineteenth-century book about sleep (from an author in St Petersburg, of all places) there was described 'a punkah-wallah who could work the punkah* with his foot fairly well while sound asleep'. Rhythmic scratching is a frequent occurrence during the unbroken sleep of those with itchy skin troubles and rhythmic tooth-grinding during sleep is even commoner.

Rhythmic movements provide their own source of sleep-promoting stimulation and when combined with the sound of rhythmic music, beating drums, clapping hands, stamping feet, and regular, rhythmic visual stimuli, as is common in the dance ceremonies of many peoples, one would anticipate a powerfully-acting trend towards lowered cortical vigilance. It does happen

---

* 'Word . . . used . . . by Anglo-Indians for a large swinging fan fixed to the ceiling and pulled by a coolie during the hot weather.' *Encyclopaedia Britannica*, 1911.

too. Some years ago I made EEG and movement recordings on volunteers while they were moving regularly to the sound of some famous dance-bands. In these investigations it was found that the brain waves would gradually alter towards those of sleep and then, especially when he felt 'sent', the dancer would continue moving rhythmically while his EEG was that of light sleep – he entered the sort of trance described by Dr William Sargant in his book *Battle for the Mind*. When this state of trance, of half-sleep, is reached in prolonged ceremonies and rituals, the individual is, of course, especially liable to see visions and hear voices.

In order to confirm that this could happen even though the eyes were open, some volunteers had their eyes stuck wide open with glue and sticking plaster, while moving their hands and legs rhythmically in time to very loud jazz music, the rhythm of which was synchronized with four strongly flashing lights in front of their eyes. The same thing resulted. What was especially significant was that, when, over and over again, for a few seconds at a time, the EEG became that of sleep and the heart rate slowed down, their movements sometimes more or less ceased. Yet afterwards they were unaware of their failures at those times. The man who, with open eyes, sits at the front of a locomotive in the presence of both rhythmic noises and regularly passing sleepers, rails, and telegraph poles, or, indeed, the man at the wheel of his car, is in a not very dissimilar situation. It is worth emphasizing that cortical vigilance, controlled by the ever-fluctuating upflow of impulses from the reticular formation, can not only vary within wide limits between day and night, but from moment to moment. You can go lightly to sleep, wake up, go to sleep and wake again within the space of a few seconds. And without realizing it.

3. Sleep is Essential

How much sleep do humans need? Left to themselves small babies sleep less than many people suppose – not twenty-odd hours but only fourteen or so. In the case of adults, it seems that there are big individual variations. One occasionally reads in the newspapers of persons who have both day-time and night-time jobs and who claim never to go to bed. One whom I encountered was a young woman who, as a child, had been taken to countless doctors by her worried parent because she simply would not sleep. Two others, both happy and healthy, regularly slept less than three hours nightly and seemed to take sleep in concentrated form, with more than expected of both the very slow EEG wave phase and of the paradoxical phase that we shall discuss later. It is not the blessing you might suppose, for it can be lonely to be awake while all around you sleep, and if you keep awakening your husband or wife just for company, the response can be disappointing. The consensus of opinion is that women seem to need more sleep on average than men, but one cannot dogmatize in the case of individuals. It is, in any event, not an easy matter to collect data which could be claimed to be free of the effects of social pressures.

The nearest approach to such freedom was available to men on an Antarctic expedition. There was non-stop daylight, the postman, milkman and newspaper-boy did not arrive at a fixed morning hour, and save that each man had his individual tasks, often requiring him to be awake at certain hours (e.g. for meteorological observations) each could sleep as he pleased. One of their little tasks, however, was to keep a careful chart of when and for how long they slept. At the end of the expedition it was found that the average charted sleep was just about the traditional eight hours.

When the sleep-pundit appears on television, the poor commentator has to think of something to say by way of introduction, and he clutches at some old saw, reminding his audience, for instance, that an hour before midnight is worth two thereafter. Obviously it is not, it all depends upon what hour you are accustomed to going to sleep. It is, however, probable that the restorative processes of sleep are at a maximum in the first couple of hours (which tend to be before midnight for many people). By some criteria sleep is deeper in the first two hours than in the last two hours. There are fewer movements and the EEG waves are bigger and slower (see p. 149).

At Edinburgh we kept six medical students awake for 108 hours. When they were finally allowed to sleep, on the first night they spent an exceptionally large part of the time with very big slow EEG waves. Such sleep-deprived people move less often too on their first night's rest. Furthermore, such people will wake after twelve to fourteen hours and feel more or less normal again that day. They may have lost four nights' sleep, but they seem to manage without ever getting an extra thirty-two hours as compensation. Which suggests that the sleep with very big slow EEG waves is an extra-potent restorative. Nevertheless, in Chapters 5 and 8 we shall see that it is not the only sleep we need.

Two other of our volunteers, for one month, lived a sort of forty-eight-hour life. They were allowed to go to bed only every other night, but, when there, were allowed to sleep as long as they liked. Gradually they got fairly accustomed to the new mode of life, until, after a month, they were thriving satisfactorily on, not sixteen hours of sleep per forty-eight, but only eleven to twelve hours' sleep. It was as if the nervous system had made adjustments so that the quality of sleep was enhanced to make up for the lack of quantity.

To spend a third of life in unproductive idleness seems a dreadful waste to some people, and now and then they decide to shun the slothful practice for evermore. No one has yet succeeded. After a couple of sleepless nights they are as sleepy as anyone else, eventually become incoherent and irrational and seek the season of all natures.

Sleep Deprivation

Many experimenters have studied sleep loss by trying totally to deprive volunteers of sleep for up to ten days and nights, or by observing men who have renounced sleep as part of a rather foolish competition. These studies have told us about the effects of acute total sleep loss, rather than the effects of chronic or long-continued restriction of the hours of sleep. We know very little about the latter other than incidentally, from observing, for example, doctors who have to work for many weeks by day and night. Irritability and a lowered resistance to infective illness seem to be common sequels.

It is very difficult to keep a volunteer from sleeping. After sixty hours or so he can slip so rapidly into sleep that he requires constant supervision. Monotony in any form speeds his passage into sleep. I have walked along the streets of Edinburgh with a sleep-deprived volunteer on either side of me and seen their eyelids closing, closing, till they walked along unseeing and in a state of light sleep. Novelty of surroundings, of company, and of activity on their part are essential for the maintenance of wakefulness. Repeatedly by day and night, one must change their activities. A walk, a game of cards, a meal, a visit to the shops, a game with dice, a shower, another short walk, making tea, finding some writing paper, buying stamps or a meeting with strangers. Without variety, sleepiness will triumph. Always one has to watch for the gently closing eyes, the sagging frame.

Something within them, perhaps a chemical build-up, is fighting against all the influences which normally excite the reticular formation, fighting to damp it down and so decrease the upflow of nerve impulses which maintain cortical vigilance or efficiency.

The EEG and other measures, such as type of movement during breathing and the exactness of eye movements, have taught us how, in a normal person, a quick drift into light sleep can last for a few seconds at a time. The liability to do so when sleep-deprived is enormously enhanced. Over and over again little 'microsleeps', as they have been called, interfere with efficient mental life and interrupt skilled behaviour.

Studying Sleepy People

How shall one demonstrate the effects of sleep loss? For many years, and not least during the years of the Second World War, when the matter seemed of practical importance, psychologists were nonplussed by the apparent lack of any effects of sleep loss on the tasks they gave to volunteers. After three days and nights without sleep the grip was as strong as before, so evidently the muscles were not fatigued. After a request to add up a list of sums, arithmetical performance seemed no worse and no better than before, so evidently the brain could still work as cleverly. Asked to respond as quickly as possible by pressing a key after a light flash which was preceded by a warning buzzer, 'reaction-time' could be as quick as ever.

The key to this puzzle has been found in latter years and is illustrated by a series of experiments carried out by a team at the Walter Reed Army Institute of Research in the U.S.A., led by a psychologist, Dr Harold Williams. They looked more carefully at the reaction-time test on sleep-deprived volunteers. Sure enough, if the volunteers were given only half a dozen reactions to make in a one-minute test they could still make instant reactions. If asked to sit and make a series of seventy-two reactions, spread irregularly over a quarter of an hour, even at the end of that time they could still make some top-speed reactions. Some. But not all. The fact that some were still top-speed showed that there was no uniformly increasing clouding of consciousness in that time. On the other hand, a close look at all the reaction-times on the days when sleep was lacking, and a comparison with performance by the same volunteers on previous days and on days following later sleep, revealed the presence of many very lengthy reaction-times scattered through the prompt ones. Furthermore, the longer the test on sleep-deprived days had lasted, the more of these long reaction-times there were. At the beginning of a reaction-time test session, most reaction-times were, as usual, about 0·3 second. By the end of the session reactions were occasionally being delayed for 1·5 or even 2·5 seconds. Moreover, this was more frequent after three days and nights without sleep than after only two days and nights.

The most reasonable interpretation of these findings was that momentary periods of sleep, 'microsleeps', were repeatedly interrupting and delaying activity, and that these became more frequent as a monotonous test session progressed, and more insistent as sleep-deprivation increased.

What about the adding-up tasks? The percentage of correct answers on sums of equal difficulty was no different on sleep-lack days than on other days. The secret lay in the time available. Given plenty of time for the arithmetic test, all was well. Told to do as many as possible in a limited time, the man short of sleep simply did not tackle as many. It looked as if he might be stopping now and then to go back and start again a sum during the middle of which he had lapsed into a microsleep.

That the latter process of having to go back and correct slips was responsible for much of the slowness was shown by teaching the volunteers a code of instructions for moving domino-like pieces to form a pattern. Then they had to speak into a tape-recorder a series of commands for the arrangement of the pieces in a complex pattern. Compared with normal days, after lacking sleep for three days, the volunteers made corrections twice as often. They made more errors but then corrected themselves, so that mere inspection of the final result would have given the impression of no impairment of their abilities.

In these and other tasks involving the solution of a series of problems, and in which the final result of the sleep-deprived man's efforts appeared no worse in quality than normal, he was allowed respite from activity. Between the warnings within each of the reaction-time test sessions, between each arithmetical sum, he could briefly relax. If allowed no respite, if required to sustain activity, if the pace of performance were imposed by some external agency or machine (as is the case in industrial conveyor-belts requiring inspection) what then would happen?

The sleep-deprived man of whom sustained attention is demanded makes frequent errors of omission and commission. He fails to do the right thing at the right time, does the right things at the wrong time or the wrong thing at any time. A simple task used by the U.S.A. research workers was one in which a series of letters from the alphabet appeared one after another. The task was simply to press a lever whenever 'X' appeared, as it did 160 times among 630 letters. This was a very easy task on which practically no errors were made when testing was carried out before and after the sleep-lack days. After three nights without sleep a quarter of the 'Xs' were missed! On the other hand, the lever was often pressed when the letter just shown had not been 'X', as if the operator suddenly realized he had just been dozing, felt sure it must have been an 'X' and hurriedly pressed the lever. It is worth emphasizing again the importance of careful experimental design in psychological experiments. In those just described, care was taken to ensure that testing before, during, and after sleep-lack days always occurred at the same hour of the day, for it was essential to rule out possible effects attributable to diurnal (or twenty-four-hour) rhythm alone.

A very similar result followed the use of a task in which the letter was not shown but spoken. Nearly forty per cent of the 'X's were missed after three nights without sleep. In this task the eyes were closed and the signs of quick little drifts into sleep were found in the EEG, associated with the apparent failures to hear the 'X's.

In the domino-like task already mentioned, when the sleep-deprived man had to issue the instructions for moving the pieces, his overall performance was perfectly sound. There he was working at his own pace. When, however, he had to listen to the instructions being given by someone else, and move the pieces about himself, he kept making serious errors, for he had no opportunity for respite or for going back and correcting what he had done wrong.

Over and over again we come up against evidence which points the same way. The sleep-deprived man can briefly be as capable as a normal one. *But he cannot sustain an effort of attention.* The challenge of a new task is accompanied, one may surmise, by a vigorous stream of nerve messages from the brain cortex down to the reticular formation ('Bestir yourself, wake me up, here's a job to be done!'). The flagging reticular formation is roused anew to excitement, so enabling peak performance to be restored. But only briefly. It cannot keep it up. Soon, lapses into drowsiness occur and mental function reveals the qualities we have discussed earlier.

One of the Edinburgh medical students, after 100 hours without sleep, was addressing a batch of envelopes from a list. One by one he was struggling through them. It was a monotonous task. Breaks began to appear in his work. Reviving, he wrote the next name, then the first part of the address, then, coming to the final line which was 'West Lothian', he wrote, 'West Looking'. He had started off all right but could not sustain his attention.

Another example illustrates the dream-like quality of thinking when cortical vigilance is lowered. When eighty hours sleepless and chatting with my colleague, Ralph Berger, about the research work, under circumstances where the phrase, 'first in the field', might have been used, the volunteer remarked, 'That is all right so long as you are first on the green'. He had a mental picture of three golf balls on a green (a 'green' not a 'field'), one being played by Berger.

These men were sometimes asked to help us by turning through the pages of some of our EEG records of all-night sleep (about a third of a mile per night). They were asked to write down the time of night on every third double page (at two-minute intervals, in fact). Another monotonous task, but one they would undertake. More intellectually-demanding tasks were anathema to them at these times. Looking through these records at their efforts one is struck by the many corrections. First 12.31, changed to 12.37 and some illegible letters after it, the whole then crossed out, 12.3 begun and crossed out, 12.30 written down and finally changed to 12.32. Sometimes, instead of times, senseless words or phrases were found to have been written, such as 'story burden' (compare with the nonsense constructions of drowsiness on p. 44), 'batting by one', 'cormial brier', 'a dorable', 'SBT', and '12.81D Cuba here we comerce'.

At times they made senseless remarks (compare again p. 44). Shortly after suddenly saying, 'Who to begin', one bent down and kissed the EEG paper. When then asked by me about this, he said he must have been dreaming about his girl-friend (who was currently denying him her hand in marriage). I asked him then to write down a description of his experience, but, once more, absurd elements quickly intruded. He wrote, 'Leant forwards and downwards to plant a kiss upon the unmaried letters. £Coo hch.' One can see the evident associations of his thought processes, EEG paper – paper letters – alphabetical – letters – hch.

Just as visions are common when falling asleep in bed, in the same way, a sleep-deprived man, forced to walk about with eyes open, often describes 'seeing things'. Surfaces of objects seem to swirl and change, the wall-paper seems to come to life, people or faces appear suddenly, only to vanish upon drawing nearer. Two of our volunteers saw crumbs on the table-cloth running about like insects. One man once spent half a minute carefully kicking at cobwebs which appeared to cover a carpet. Three had visions of women peering at them. One saw them in broad daylight, almost always unpleasant old women, who appeared to be talking about him. They would vanish Cheshire-cat-wise, the body before the face, as he drew near, but after passing he saw them again when he turned round!

'Hearing things' too is quite common: dogs barking, voices speaking amidst the noise of running water. Longer and more pervasive dream states interfere with ordinary conversation, quite irrelevant replies or remarks being made which seem to refer to a vivid day-dream life rather than to real life.

Most striking is the unpleasant, nightmare-like day-dream life into which some fall. Many teams of experimenters have seen this in a few of their volunteers. Oblique remarks and veiled hints begin to be made, to indicate that a new understanding has dawned of how some organization, or the experimenters, are engaged upon some secret and harmful plot. Into these obtrudes the sort of thinking that we have seen before – one of our volunteers referred to Ralph Berger as an 'exquisitor' to indicate an inquisitor able to inflict exquisite pain. Another volunteer, whom we shall call Arthur, on his fourth day since last sleeping, entered a paranoid state of a kind which illustrates what other experimenters too have observed.

He was in company with another volunteer, whom we shall call Sandy. They were being supervised during the day by me.

In the mid-morning we had coffee before going off on a shopping expedition. Walking along a main street, Arthur walked behind Sandy, bending forwards, peering and pointing at the latter's jacket. He said he saw handwriting on it. A few minutes later he insisted on his companion taking off his jacket in the street (which he did) for closer inspection. I explained to him that 'seeing things' was common during sleep-deprivation, but from then on he built up an elaborate system of delusions which he did not divulge till seven hours later and not fully till the next day, when, after sleep, he wrote nine pages of description.

It had been arranged that he and his companion should appear on television that evening. He began to think he must have been given a drug in order that he should have something interesting to recount on television. He remembered having been told to drink up his morning coffee before the shopping expedition and decided the drug must have been put into the coffee. At lunch:

We were put at a table well away from the rest . . . I said, 'What do they think we are, bloody pariahs?' I then thought I heard someone two or three tables away talking about the word pariah and its derivation. I decided I must have been treated so that although I thought I spoke in a normal voice I was, in fact, shouting. During the afternoon I was doubtful what I should do about this information I had as I didn't want to tell —.

He was driven with Berger and Sandy to Glasgow in a television company car. Arthur felt frightened, for Berger was questioning Sandy about his dreams, and slowly the realization dawned that Berger was taking Sandy away to lock him up after first hypnotizing him, for Sandy kept crossing and uncrossing his legs at Berger's command (actually this was to help keep Sandy awake). A word-game, too, was played to help maintain alertness, but Arthur (as he later wrote) 'was very wary of this' because of the danger of saying a significant word, like a Freudian slip of the tongue (which is supposed to indicate your unconscious hidden desires). When given the word, 'train', he replied, 'Glasgow', for it instantly dawned on him that Sandy must be about to be locked up for having been responsible for fires on the Glasgow blue electric trains withdrawn from service some months before. Then came the realization that it was he, not Sandy, who must be about to be locked up. He became frightened. Berger noticed the strange, fixed stare on his face and received a large number of evasive and queer replies to questions ('discovering the unknown'; 'the guilty one'; 'the characters are different'). They reached the television studios, which Arthur took to be a hospital. He then confessed his fears and beliefs, was taken indoors and, when shown the cameras, etc., seemed reassured. After a night's sleep he was restored to normal.

The irrational thinking of sleep-deprived persons, exemplified by Arthur, resembles that of certain mental illnesses, notably paranoid schizophrenia. At the present time a good deal of research (though not nearly enough, considering the commonness of that illness) is devoted to exploring possible abnormalities of brain chemical function in schizophrenia. One approach has been to give drugs like mescaline and lysergic acid diethylamide (LSD 25) to volunteers and study the resulting states of intoxication which in some respects resemble schizophrenia. They are, incidentally, much enhanced by sleep-deprivation. This has been with a view to pursuing related chemical compounds to see if these might produce even more typically schizophrenic states, and, of course, to try and discover whether chemicals of this kind exist in the brain.

Persuasion and False Confession

The brain of the sleep-deprived person just is not capable of sustaining normal levels of efficiency. If we carry out EEG examinations at such times we find that the volunteers will do simple tasks, and answer questions which require no great feats of comprehension, while the EEG rhythms are those of drowsiness or light sleep. An important consequence of lowered cortical vigilance, or efficiency, is a relative inability simultaneously to relate data from a variety of sources, especially to bring to bear upon present problems information gained in the past. This has been demonstrated in the laboratory by giving sleep-deprived people problems to solve, the solution of which would have been aided had they remembered what they had had the opportunity of learning in times past. Their capacity to bring the past to bear upon their present problems was abnormally poor. Of more general interest, however, is the political prisoner under pressure to agree to a new philosophy, to renounce what he had learned in the past, even to denounce his past activities in lurid or false terms, to forget the past hostility and vices of his interrogators and to embrace them as his true friends.

During the Korean War, airmen of the U.S.A. who had become prisoners of the Chinese confessed to having dropped germs upon their foes. They were eventually repatriated. The U.S.A. authorities were naturally very concerned about these false confessions, and intensive studies were made of the re-patriated airmen, and diligent inquiries directed to all other possible sources concerning the conditions which led up to the false confessions. These conditions have been described in a number of reports, such as R. J. Lifton's very readable *Thought Reform and the Psychology of Totalism*. A feature of these Chinese and other 'brain-washing' procedures (as American journalists chose to call them) was sleep-deprivation. The victim was deliberately kept awake by a succession of guards, interrogated at night when normal diurnal rhythms favoured lowered cortical vigilance, and subjected to an endlessly repeated series of questions and arguments. Subjected, in other words, to mono-tony in a situation of constant threat. Normally a threatening situation causes arousal and not sleepiness. If the threat is over-whelming, or if combined with physical restraint, as with prisoners, a sleep state results (see Chapter 6). Furthermore, a constantly, monotonously, repeated threat, when it finally leads to breakdown of the arousal or awakening mechanisms, is followed by a more total state of inertness than a monotonously repeated stimulus of lesser significance (see p. 112).

Interrogation of this kind is often a sequel to prolonged total isolation. In Canada, experiments have shown that volunteers subjected to prolonged isolation and lack of normal, varied stimulation of sight, touch and hearing, not only sometimes develop false perceptions – 'seeing things', for example – but, as the days pass, have a slowing down of the EEG rhythms similar to that of drowsiness. The really remarkable thing is that, after isolation of this kind for a couple of weeks, the brain rhythms refuse to accelerate to normal again for up to a week or more after release, while behaviourally the men lack initiative and energy.

It is apparent that, under what may be called conventional brain-washing conditions, the physiological state of the brain might be expected to be so altered that efficiency would be reduced, grasp of former realities would be impaired, and thoughts, words, actions and beliefs might be accepted that would previously have been rejected as incompatible with the established facts of past reality.

But It's Nicer to Stay in Bed

In medical practice one encounters occasional patients who sleep too much. Some of these hypersomniacs remain sluggish and unable to concentrate for half an hour or more after waking. Can normal people have too much of a good thing? Most of us are accustomed to having our eight hours and then leaping out of bed eager to meet the day. Suppose, however, we were people who had the capacity to sleep for a longer period and, once in a while, were permitted to sleep on for eleven hours. Being even more rested, should we then be even more alert in our performance? In order to test the statement sometimes heard that excess sleep produces a feeling of grogginess, Ralph Berger (by now resident in sunny California), with the help of a student, let six volunteers sleep eight hours on one night and eleven hours on the next, while another six slept eleven hours on their first night and eight hours the next. Half an hour after awakening each morning and at the same hour of day they were required to sustain a high level of attention for fifteen minutes, just like the sleep-deprived men on p. 54. They had to try and spot which few out of a long series of doorbell buzzes, occurring once every two and a half seconds, were six-tenths instead of only four-tenths of a second long. After eleven hours' sleep the men spotted fewer of the long buzzes and more often wrongly thought a short buzz was a long one than was the case after eight hours of sleep. The then student, Taub, has gone on in more recent years to amplify and confirm this work and it has become plain that, while prolonged sleep deprivation is the worst enemy of efficiency, any departure from the usual routine of sleep, whether in duration or timing, is associated with impairment of performance.

4. New Light on Dreaming

Most people believe they dream for a few minutes most nights. Others will say they never dream. At the end of the last century psychologists discovered that, if they awakened themselves by alarm clocks during the night, they found more often than expected that they had just been dreaming, especially if the awakening was delayed till the later hours of sleep. Earlier in this book we have noted how sleep seems to prevent the formation of clear memories. As we shall see, this applies strikingly to dreams, nearly all of which are forgotten practically at once.

What do we mean by a dream? Dreams are sometimes defined as a succession of visual images or mental pictures. I believe this is misleading. True enough, people will say, 'I saw a huge bus coming towards me in a dream'. But it was not just a moving picture of a bus. It was experienced as something having a vivid personal reference, coming 'towards me', in a situation where the 'me' was then not in real time but in dream-time. A little further questioning will reveal that the individual was dreaming that he was, perhaps, on his bicycle at the time, in some far away and vaguely recognized city, at some point of earlier life. In reality he was simply in bed. But he was experiencing the adventure of an unreal life, a dream-life or fantasy-life, in which he was far removed from his downy pillow. A dream is part of a fantasy life. As in real life things are seen in it. So too sounds are heard, conversations conducted, people are met, some of whom are felt to be friendly and some hostile, things are done, fear and joy are felt.

It may make things clearer if we consider the case of men blind from birth. They dream. Of course they cannot see things in their dreams because they have no conception of what seeing is. (Try explaining to such a man what the colour 'red' looks like.) Just as in real life they meet people, hear things, feel things, smell things, do things, so too in their dreams they meet people, hear, feel, smell and do things. But they do not see things. When I once woke up a man who had always been blind he described his dream. How he had been in the Blind Workshop with a friend. How they had put a rosary into a football so that they should hear it when they kicked it. They had not really; he had been lying asleep in a laboratory. He had been dreaming.

We have already considered how, when people are drowsy after settling to sleep in bed, the quality of their mental life soon changes. Contact with reality becomes gradually more and more tenuous and, if then roused, many people will describe having just had dream experiences in some setting far from their quiet beds. Their day-dreams had passed on to and merged into night-dreams. This had happened when the EEG lost its alpha rhythm and a pattern of low voltage slow waves was present. However, we now know that normal people do most of their dreaming much later in the night; that there may be as much as one and a half or two hours of dreaming; and that at those times the EEG resembles in appearance the EEG of drowsiness (though, as we shall see, resemblance in the function of other parts of the body is much less). How did this come to be discovered?

The story begins during the early 1950s in Chicago with Dr Nathaniel Kleitman and a research student of his, now Dr Aserinsky. They were studying the sleep of infants in the first months of life and making continuous round-the-clock observations. They noticed that there was a recurrent or cyclical pattern of restlessness, a cycle having an hourly periodicity. Every hour too, the infants' eyes moved about for a few minutes beneath the closed lids. Would a similar periodic change in sleep be found in adults? They set to work to find out.

Wires from the EEG machine were attached to the scalp and face of volunteers. It can easily be arranged for these to be so comfortable that they become unnoticed: little silver discs and a spot of salty jelly make contact between the skin and the wire, the discs being held in place with adhesive plaster on the face and with glue on the scalp. Kleitman and his colleagues – Kleitman was joined by a tremendously energetic medical student, now Dr Bill Dement – used the wires going to the face to pick up sudden changes of electrical potential caused by movements of the eyeballs. At rest there is always a difference in potential between the outside and the deep interior of the eye, and when the eyeballs swing round the EEG machine very easily picks up evidence of the alteration of the position of the two zones of the eyeball.

They found that a recurrent or cyclical pattern could be seen in the sleep of adults, just as in the sleep of infants. Instead of an hourly periodicity, in adults the changes showed up about every one and a half hours. As the volunteer fell asleep in the bedroom adjacent to the EEG laboratory, alpha rhythm disappeared from his EEG (Figure 1) and his eyeballs made gently rolling, slow movements. Then within a few minutes the eyes became still, and sleep spindles made their appearance. Gradually the EEG waves got bigger and bigger, slower and slower, with little bursts of spindles (Figure 1). But then, for a period of some minutes, the picture would change, the EEG became one of low voltage and the eyes made frequent jerky, rapid movements. The two eyes moved together or 'conjugately', as in waking life. Four, five or six of these rapid eye movement periods were present in each night.

Could it be, they thought, that these rapid eye movements are an indication of the dreamer 'looking around' at the visual events of his dream-world? To find out they worked night after night, waking up their volunteers, sometimes from the rapid eye movement periods, sometimes from the sleep in which the eyes were still and the EEG waves large and slow. Watching, hour by hour, the tireless pens of the EEG machine, they could make an alarm ring in the bedroom at whatever phase of sleep they chose. Using a two-way microphone and loudspeaker system, with a tape-recorder, they would ask, 'Have you been dreaming?' 'No, I wasn't', would come the reply when awakenings were made from sleep with big, slow EEG waves and spindles, from the periods when the eyes were not moving. 'Yes, yes, I was dreaming, I was dreaming I was going with my friend to the . . .' – a long dream description, when awakened from a rapid eye movement period.

After 351 awakenings they found that on eighty per cent of occasions dreams had been described after awakening from rapid eye movement periods, but only seven per cent after the other awakenings. Furthermore, those seven per cent were only fragmentary memories compared with the lengthy narratives from rapid eye movement period awakenings. What is more, the length of the narrative was roughly proportional to the length of time the sleeper had been allowed to go on with his rapid eye movement period before being awakened. If he had been awakened after only ten minutes from the start of such a period, the adventures described were of a kind that would have occupied about ten minutes in real life. If he had been awakened after twenty minutes, the adventures were of a kind that would have occupied about twenty minutes in real life. The conclusions were both inescapable and novel: dreaming recurs several times each night in normal people even if they cannot remember it in the morning; dreaming is an affair extended in time rather than a matter of brief flashes.

A team of research workers in New York learned of the Chicago experiments and felt sceptical. They then set out to test the Chicago claims for themselves. What of people claiming never to dream? From a large number of volunteers they selected one group of those who said they were frequent dreamers, and a second group of those who thought they never dreamed. Their volunteers' all-night sleep was watched over, they too were wakened, sometimes from periods of sleep with motionless eyes and EEG big slow waves and sleep spindles, and sometimes from rapid eye movement periods. The 'dreamers' reported dreams after fifty-three and ninety-three per cent of these awakenings respectively, the 'non-dreamers' after seventeen and forty-six per cent respectively. The differences between the two classes of awakenings were much greater than could be ascribed to chance alone, as were the differences between the 'dreamers' and 'non-dreamers'. The experimenters had found the same sort of cyclical pattern in all-night sleep as the Chicago workers. Now thoroughly convinced, the New Yorkers proposed that the fairly high incidence of dream reports from sleep with motion-less eyes could well be attributed to recall of what had been dreamed in a prior rapid eye movement period.

A most important point was stressed by these experimenters. What is it that is called 'a dream'? People who said they never dreamed were not just people who seemed to forget their dreams almost at once, they were often people for whom a dream had to be something quite bizarre or crazy. The individual might say that, no, he had not been dreaming, he had only been 'thinking'. He might say he had been 'thinking' he was riding in a motor-car with his friend and they were just passing a large yellow lorry, when all the time he was actually lying in bed. He did not call the vivid fantasy-adventure in which he was living a dream, because it was internally consistent. To him a 'dream' meant something made up of crazy elements.

The essential findings made by the Chicago pioneers have been confirmed in laboratories all over the world and have led to further discoveries, the University of Chicago retaining an honourable position among the leaders. One of the subsequent experiments carried out there reveals most clearly the rapidity with which dreams are forgotten. Ten volunteers were awakened in the course of fifty-one nights during, and at different times after the end of, rapid eye movement periods. When wakened from a rapid eye movement period, on forty-six out of fifty-four occasions, dream descriptions which could be classified as 'detailed' were obtained. When wakened five minutes after the end of a rapid eye movement period, no detailed dream reports were given, although on nine of the eleven occasions 'fragments' were recalled. When wakened ten or more minutes after the end of a rapid eye movement period, there was one dream fragment from twenty-six occasions, there being no dream-recall at all after the other twenty-five.

Variations in frequency of dream-recall could depend partly on differences in remembering power, and perhaps partly on some enthusiastic volunteers unwittingly embellishing their re-ports while giving them. Also on the general level of motivation, intellect and cooperation. There is a brain operation, called modified leucotomy, which is occasionally done to alleviate very severe mental suffering when all else has failed, especially when the patient is tormented by constant self-questioning. After this operation had been practised for ten years or so, reports began to appear to the effect that, after it, people did not dream. Here we see a good illustration of the change of standards that has now to be applied when considering the merits of statements about dreaming. The conclusions about leucotomized patients were reached after some of these patients had been asked at day-time interviews whether they could remember dreaming since the operation.

Today we have to apply quite different standards of critical appraisal. We now know that normal people only remember an insignificant fraction of their total dreams. A claim that dreaming is abolished by operation would now require laboratory studies of all-night sleep and awakenings from sleep. When this is actually done, cyclically recurring rapid eye movement periods are still found to be present after leucotomy, and when awakened from these, dreaming is reported. But one effect of leucotomy is to reduce the degree of lively interest in helping others that a normal person will display. Woken up from slumber by investigating doctors, the leutocomized patient simply does not bother to pause and let the memory of the dream come back in detail. He snorts affirmatively that he was indeed dreaming, describes in a few words 'where' he was in his dreams and promptly turns over, determined to get back to sleep at once.

When Do We Dream?

Are we to conclude that dreaming is confined to the rapid eye movement periods? At the time of writing the general opinion would, I think, be that vivid, adventurous dreams are most often contemporary with rapid eye movement periods, but that dreams no less vivid and adventurous are sometimes experienced when first falling asleep and that mental life during sleep is by no means confined to rapid eye movement periods but can occur at any time of the night.

In Chapter 1 I described experiments which showed that the sleeping brain could discriminate between meaningful and meaningless noises, between words issuing backwards from a tape-recorder and the same words played normally. This was true of sleep when the eyes were motionless and the EEG waves very large and slow, so that what we normally consider as mental function was not wholly absent at those times. Furthermore, people talk in their sleep. Curiously enough, there are very great individual differences in this respect. Some people talk much more than others. Sometimes they talk in the course of a rapid eye movement period. More often sleep-talking accompanies a general bodily stirring which interrupts the other phase of sleep, the phase in which the eyes are quiescent and the EEG waves large and slow. In the latter case, an American study of people who sleep-talked revealed that the content of what was spoken often pertained to the laboratory situation, tended to be un-emotional, and only sometimes related to a little mental content recalled upon deliberately rousing the sleeper and questioning him. By contrast, they found that the words spoken during a rapid eye movement period often were emotionally charged, and were clearly related to the dream described on subsequently rousing the sleeper. Nevertheless it must be noted that *some* mental life was said to have been present when the eyes were quiescent and the EEG waves large and slow.

Another source of evidence is provided by the sleep rockers and rollers I mentioned in Chapter 2. Quite common among very small children, this rhythmic movement at night is much less common among older children, although, among the latter, it is more frequent if there is also blindness or if the child has lived in an institution. I have been able to study two youths, one of thirteen and one of twenty, who, physically and psychologi-cally, were otherwise normal. I have never witnessed such an extraordinary spectacle as that presented by the large twenty-year-old man. Lying peacefully asleep this huge fellow would abruptly and violently fling his head and body rhythmically to left and right. The thirteen-year-old would suddenly turn on to his hands and knees and hurl his head rhythmically at the pillow ... bang ... bang ... bang ... bang. There would be a dozen or a hundred of the movements before they ceased. Then sleep would continue as if nothing had happened. Each made the movements at the rate of one per second. I tried doing the same myself one day and found that to exceed a rate of one movement per one and a half seconds was extremely difficult.

In order to study the sleep of these young men, wires from the EEG machine were attached to their faces and scalps, while others were placed on some of the body muscles to get a direct record of movement. In addition, strong steel wires passing through the mattress were disturbed by any big movement and pulled on bent steel rulers at the foot of the bed. What are known as 'strain gauges', which had been stuck on to the rulers, were used to provide a record of the bending and unbending of the rulers, and so of the mattress movements, concurrently with the records direct from the individual's body.

I had thought that, probably, these movements would begin after a brief period of wakefulness in the middle of the night, a kind of sleepy attempt at rocking oneself off to deeper sleep, baby-fashion. But this surmise proved quite wrong. The rocking movements began abruptly during sleep and were not accompanied by signs of awakening. Most commonly they began during a rapid eye movement period. But sometimes they began during sleep with motionless eyes and large EEG slow waves and sleep spindles.

The rocking in infancy (and these men had done it since infancy) is a comfort response of young primates – monkeys, chimpanzees, humans – to loneliness and fear. One could therefore regard the rocking during the rapid eye movement periods as a response to an unhappy dream. The fact that it sometimes occurred at other times in the night makes one suspect that at any hour of the night some sort of mental life can be present, and that, in these young men, it was sometimes an unhappy form of mental life; mental life of a kind from which, long ago, they had learned to seek relief in rhythmic movement.

Another approach to this question of the presence of mental life in different stages of sleep was adopted by Dr David Foulkes in Chicago. Whereas, in the pioneer experiments, volunteers were wakened and asked whether they had been dreaming, Foulkes asked his volunteers, 'Was anything passing through your mind?' This difference in the form of the question elicited results strikingly different from those of the earlier experimenters. Rapid eye movement awakenings elicited reports of mental experience just beforehand on eighty-seven per cent of occasions. Awakenings from the other phase of sleep, when the eyes were motionless, elicited reports on seventy per cent of occasions. Foulkes went further and carefully analysed the actual content of the description. How much visual imagery? How much emotion? Movement and 'scene' shifts? And so on. There was some overlap in the quality of the descriptions, but what his study revealed very clearly was that, compared with the other awakenings, when awakened from rapid eye movement periods a person was more likely to describe 'dreaming' than 'thinking', more likely to describe vivid adventures spiced with imagery, action and emotion, in settings far removed in space and time from the laboratory. Awakenings from sleep with motionless eyes more often produced reports of having been 'thinking' about mundane events of the previous day.

The objection can be made, and has by some authors, that reports of mental life upon awakening from sleep might be simply memories of what was going through the mind when first falling asleep, or might be formed during the moments of actual waking-up. The evidence about the relation between length of dream narrative and duration of preceding rapid eye movement period, the relation of the content of the dream to outside events and to the number of eye movements (see below) and the difference between the reports from the two phases of sleep, makes this an implausible explanation of recall after rapid eye movement awakenings. It does, however, offer an explanation of the 'thinking' about current events in Foulkes's study of awakenings from sleep with motionless eyes. Inferences already made about the night rockers and rollers, and similar inferences we shall make about sleep-walkers (p. 94), offer evidence of mental life at those times which cannot be so readily explained away.

In Figure 6 there is an illustration of a psycho-galvanic response. These responses, or sudden changes in the spontaneous electrical potential at the palm (which can also be found by recording skin electrical conductivity), occur during wakefulness after a sudden emotional stimulus, but they also appear spontaneously, and then their abundance during wakefulness is believed to be an indication of recurrent anxious feelings. In the experiments which were illustrated in Figure 6 we noticed that when some volunteers passed into what we believed to be very deep sleep, with continuous very large and very slow EEG waves, spontaneous skin potential changes which looked like psycho-galvanic responses were traced out ceaselessly. In jocular vein, and supposing that inhibitions somehow housed in the brain cortex could be thought of as removed in this state of sleep, I took a leaf from Freud's book and referred to these skin electrical storms (as others have since called them) as displaying 'the id rampant'.

We had no idea what they really meant. In Oklahoma, however, research workers have since found that these skin electrical storms during sleep are greater if the day has been an anxious one, and both at Oklahoma and at Edinburgh we have found that ordinary sleeping pills, which will reduce anxiety, reduce the skin potentials in sleep with large slow EEG waves. Psycho-galvanic responses by day certainly are linked with anxious thoughts and feelings. It seems plausible that in sleep they may still be a sign of primitive mental life having similar qualities.

In short, I believe that some sort of mental life can probably go on all through the night, that it is almost entirely forgotten, but that it has special qualities during the phase accompanied by rapid eye movements, qualities which are those of 'dreaming'.

The Eye Movements and Other Bodily Changes

Kleitman and his co-workers suggested that the rapid eye movements were looking-at-the-dream-picture movements. What evidence is there for and against this? At the same time as the rapid eye movements, facial twitches occur in humans, but even more in chimpanzees. Are these grimacing-at-the-dream-situation twitches? Or do both happen to accompany, or to be an expression of, the total condition of the nervous system which prevails at these times (see Chapter 5) irrespective of accompanying mental life?

The American workers looked at their electrical records of the moments just before awakening and noted the direction of the last eye movement in each case. They questioned the speaker about the last event of the dream and guessed at the probable last direction of eye movement that would have accompanied such an event in real life. There was a remarkably close concordance between these directions.

The Chicago workers also scored the electrical records of the dreams of each eye movement period as 'active' and 'passive' depending on the profusion of movements, and reported that this was related to the nature of the dream content. Watching lawn tennis in real life would involve lots of eye movements, whereas sitting and watching a television screen would involve few eye movements. A dream of the former would be 'active', a dream of the latter 'passive'. In these experiments the same experimenters made subjective judgements about both the electrical records and the dreams. It could be objected that unwitting subjective bias might have crept in. Their findings therefore stood in need of confirmation by others.

At Edinburgh we took an opportunity to subject the claims about active and passive dreams to further and rigorous examination. Ralph Berger had been doing some experiments (of which more on p. 80) in which he woke people up at night from their dreams and tape-recorded their descriptions. I had never been there on those nights. The first important thing about this arrangement was that I did not get too tired! But secondly, that I did not know which dream description followed which electrical record and was therefore an independent judge. Berger gave me the eighty-nine tape-recorded dreams and I classed each as 'active' or 'passive' according to the nature of the events described, and whether or not they would have been accompanied by many shifts of gaze had they occurred in real life.

Subsequently Berger wrote code numbers on each electrical record to make sure I could not identify the individual from whom it was derived. I classified each rapid eye movement period as 'active' or 'passive' according to the profusion of eye movements during it. Some dreams only had a few isolated eye movements per minute. During others the eyes would thrash hither and thither twenty times within a few seconds, a tumult of activity. After the first scoring the records were all shuffled and I scored them again. Then, wherever there was divergence between my first and second score, Berger took out the record, put it in a new pile and re-shuffled. A final and deciding judgement was then made so that eventually every record had been given a consistent score twice out of three times.

After all this had been done the code was broken, and the judgement, 'active' or 'passive', for each electrical record of eye movements was compared with the judgement made for its respective dream. It may be added that I had been very sceptical of any association between 'active' dreams and 'active' eye movement records. I was decisively shown the need to revise my views. Fifty dreams had been judged 'active', and of these forty-two had been described after eye movement periods judged 'active'. With the thirty-nine 'passive' dreams the balance was the other way, twenty-three being related in time to 'passive' eye movement records and only sixteen to records in which eye movements were judged more profuse. Not an absolute one-to-one association, but that is not what the biologist expects. He expects to have to use simple mathematical procedures to assess his data. The statistical calculations showed that the degree of association between the nature of the dream content and the contemporaneous profusion of eye movements that we had found would be expected to arise by chance alone less often than once in a thousand times. In other words, it could not reasonably be attributed to chance. The actual numbers in the different categories of this study were in fact very close to those in the original report by Drs Dement and Wolpert of Chicago, and the small problem may serve as an example of the manner in which research makes its steady progress by way of discovery and confirmation.

In some early New York experiments the story of each dream prior to awakenings was studied and predictions were made of the direction and frequency of eye movements which could have been recorded in the half minute before the awakening had the dream events been real life events. Many of the electrical records of actual eye movements were found to show a remarkable concordance. The snag, however, was that the judgement of concordance had not been made 'blind' and when, some years later, Berger carried out similar experiments, with full precautions against unwitting bias, no concordance showed up to strengthen the looking-at-the-dream-pictures theory.

But could there not be another explanation? Could it not be that sometimes the brain is generally active, and at other times, whether in response to a drug or not, generally more quiescent? Might not some diffuse 'invigorating' influence cause active dreams and, independently, lots of eye movements? This possibility cannot be denied. In support of the alternative explanation can be cited the fact that the eye movements tend to occur in clusters or groups separated by relatively inactive periods of several seconds. In many people a few easily recognizable EEG waves of special appearance, called 'saw-toothed' waves, precede each of the clusters of eye movements. In other words, something special is happening in the brain for several seconds before the eyes move. If the eye movements were 'looking' responses to the dream events, and if dreams occur as continuous programmes rather than as sudden flashes (an old idea rejected by the American researchers) the sequence of brain waves before eye movements is hard to explain. If the brain waves simply denote a recurrent change in the electrical *status quo* of the brain, then the eye movements can be seen as a sequel.

An obvious way to check on the looking-at-dream-pictures theory was to study blind men. I was sceptical of the theory and was fairly sure men blind from birth, who could not 'see' things in their dreams, would have rapid eye movements like other people, and so set about scouring Edinburgh to find willing volunteers. It was not every blind man who was willing to go off with a stranger to sleep in the mental hospital where our laboratory was situated. The sequence of observations and interpretations provide a cautionary tale.

Three men blind for three, ten and fifteen years, respectively, said they could still picture things in their minds by day and that they still saw things in their dreams. They had rapid eye movements at night. Nothing very surprising in that. Three men blind all their lives, whose eyeballs moved freely as a movement reflex when they turned over in bed, and who, naturally, could not picture things, still had the cyclically recurring changes in the appearance of the EEG through the night. When wakened from the low voltage EEG periods they described dreaming just as normal people do. Unlike normal people, the low voltage EEG was not accompanied by rapid eye movements.

It certainly seemed that the blind men were on the side of the American theory. But how easily one can make wrong interpretations. We had used our normal technique for recording eye movements, whereby silver disc electrodes on the face pick up electrical potentials caused by eyeball movements. But what we had not realized was that those potentials depend upon a healthy retina and that in some blind men the retina has deteriorated so much that, even though their eyes move, no potentials can be picked up. Dr Charles Fisher and his colleagues in New York have used a sensitive device on the eyelids to tell them when the eyes moved and they have found rapid eye movements in men blind all their lives. So, having for several years believed my original scepticism not to have been justified, I must now admit that men blind all their lives, who do not 'see' in their dreams, probably do still have rapid eye movements and that these cannot be looking-at-the-dream-picture movements, any more than similar eye movements in the sleep of newborn babies. It is impossible to expect babies to organize a dream life, full of visual incidents, for they can have no memories round which to build such dreams. Moreover many of the eye movements of adults are rotatory movements and quite unlike those made in looking at things in real life. It remains possible that occasional large eye movements during a dream may be a manifestation of active participation, of really looking towards some dream object, but in general the eye movements are not looking-at-the-dream movements, but are signs of brain excitement and profuse eye movements mean a high level of brain excitement, reflected also in exciting dreams.

In fact Foulkes, with Molinari from Italy, has now shown that dream-life between eye movement bursts is like that in sleep with big, slow EEG waves and motionless eyes, whereas awakenings *just after* a burst of eye movements indicate that the vivid visual experiences traditional to dreaming *have just been* experienced.

We now have other instances of bodily functions which vary in intensity with the intensity of the dream experience (see also p. 93). When we are frightened adrenalin pours out into our blood and this changes some of the fat in our tissues into free fatty acids in the blood. In Cincinnati, volunteers slept while fine tubes passed from an arm vein to equipment in which the blood could be analysed whenever necessary. They were awakened near the end of their rapid eye movement periods and their dreams were tape-recorded. The dreams were then studied by people who knew nothing about the blood. They rated the dreams as calm dreams, anxious dreams or very anxious dreams. The higher the level of anxiety betrayed in the dream, the greater the rise of the 'free fatty acids' in the blood between the time of starting the rapid eye movement period and the time of the awakening from the dream. Presumably dream anxiety, like waking anxiety, causes adrenalin release.

Adrenalin makes the heart work more forcefully and, if the heart's arteries are not in good condition, such forceful work can cause an attack of angina, namely pain coming from the heart. People with narrowing of the coronary arteries to the heart muscles often get this pain when they exercise vigorously, or get cold or anxious. Sometimes they wake up suddenly from sleep with their pain, and we now know that they will do so especially often from rapid eye movement periods, as if a dream may have been responsible for an outpouring of adrenalin.

Men with duodenal ulcers also often wake up from sleep with their ulcer pain. If they sip a little milk the pain goes away, and they can sleep once more. The milk helps because it neutralizes stomach acids which cause the pain. These stomach acids increase in people with ulcers whenever there is a rapid eye movement period, though whether they do so more when the dream is an anxious one is not certain.

Dream Modification

The fact that one may now be sure that a person is dreaming at any given moment has made practicable attempts to influence the course of a dream by some outside stimulus. The Chicago workers tried the effect of light flashes, musical notes and even a water spray! Shortly afterwards they would wake up the dreamer using a bell, and inquire about his dream. On a proportion of occasions there did seem to be a connection between what was described and the outside stimulus. This was especially so with the water spray, which seemed to provoke the appearance of a sudden rain shower in the dream! The awakening bell too was sometimes incorporated into the dream-life. As a telephone bell, for example. On one occasion the dreamer was in a house when he experienced the sound of the doorbell. He was asked to answer it. He hesitated, then started to go, whereupon it rang again. In fact, the experimenter's finger had slipped off the bell-push so that he inadvertently caused it to ring twice. The interval had been one of three or four seconds. Since, in the dream, the interval between the two bells had only been very short compared with the duration of the whole dream, substance was added to the belief that long dream sequences are not experienced in a flash of time.

Some more refined experiments were undertaken in Edinburgh by my colleague Ralph Berger, whose experimental design avoided the danger that apparent modification of the dream might be ascribed only to the bias of a judge who already knew about the nature of the stimulus used during the dream. His studies also reveal very clearly the devious manner in which the mind works during dreams. It is a manner reminiscent of the mental illness schizophrenia. Reminiscent too of the curious thinking processes in drowsiness, at which time the EEG, though not quite identical, has many similarities to that present during rapid eye movement periods.

Male and female Edinburgh University student volunteers were used. Each was interviewed and a life history obtained, including their past and present romantic attachments. A specious reason being given, to the effect that their emotionality was being tested, each sat through readings of a long list of words, including the names of the past or present boy- and girl-friends, mixed with a lot of other 'neutral' names. While this was being done, their psycho-galvanic responses (p. 34) were recorded from the skin of the palm of the hand. Not surprisingly, the name of a current or past girl-friend would cause a big psycho-galvanic response. The person concerned is wholly unaware of this response (which is also used in the unreliable 'lie-detector' test). Many of the 'neutral' names caused no galvanic skin responses. For each girl volunteer Berger chose two 'neutral' boys' names and two names of boy-friends which gave rise to big psycho-galvanic responses, and vice versa for the men. Four stimulus names for each volunteer.

As a precaution against unwitting over-cooperation, the volunteers were all deliberately misled about the purpose of the experiments. They were not told, and did not discover, that name stimuli were going to be played from a loudspeaker while they were asleep and dreaming. But if noises were made in the room would they not awaken? Yes, they would, and at first they did. The first experiments were 'pilot' experiments. 'Pilot' experiments are a vital first step in almost any research programme. No matter how cleverly one thinks one has designed an experiment, things always go wrong when it comes to translating theory into practice. Only by practical experience of a new technique are the snags revealed and a satisfactory technique evolved.

Berger therefore eventually got volunteers to fall asleep against a background of 'white' noise, noise of all frequencies, like the rushing and roaring of a waterfall, varying all the time in loudness. Having got used to a constant din, the dreamer did not awaken when new sounds, spoken names from a tape recorder, were added. The name *Morag* had been played while a pilot volunteer was dreaming. Later he described dreaming of being on a *moor*, it was 'connected' with the *war*. It looked as if the sound of a stimulus might cause similar-sounding, or assonant, content-change in the dream. Having ironed out lots of other little snags, especially apparatus that at first had proved temperamental, all was set for the main experiment.

On thirty-seven nights, spread out over several months,

Berger woke up volunteers from rapid eye movement periods on 103 occasions. Eighty-nine worthwhile dream descriptions were recorded on tape – a very similar percentage to that in the original Chicago experiments. During each dreaming period Berger played a name at intervals of a few seconds. Only one name was used for each dream, but each volunteer had about ten dreams in all, and four different names were used with each person – some names during one dream only, others being played during three different dreams. None of the volunteers realized what was actually going on in the experiment and when, some months later, its true nature was divulged to them they were very surprised.

How to assess the dream descriptions? Obviously Berger himself could not do this, for, knowing the nature of the stimulus in each case, he would be tempted to see connections somewhere in the long dream narratives, connections which would be apparent and not real connections, connections which should be attributed to chance alone. It was necessary, therefore, that someone else should look for connections between the stimulus name and the dream description, someone who could not know which name had been played during which dream. If he could connect an individual name with an individual dream fairly often, the odds against his choosing so well by chance alone could then be calculated.

Berger gave me the dream descriptions. I had never been present on the experimental nights. Each volunteer's dreams, about ten of them, were given me at a time, together with the four names played during their dreams. I had to guess from studying the dream descriptions, which name went with which dream. Sometimes it was only a matter of guessing, but with others there seemed a fairly close connection between the name and the dream. When, finally, Berger added up all my choices, he found I had guessed right on thirty-two of the eighty-nine occasions. This may not seem a very high success rate till you remember that, by chance alone, I should have made the correct choice once in four times, that is to say, twenty-two or twenty-three times. When dealing with fairly large numbers, so big a discrepancy from chance makes it look as if some other factor was guiding the choices, and calculation showed that only once in two hundred times would chance alone give so good a score. In psychological experiments that is generally as much as one can say. One has to express one's finding in terms of statistics, in terms of likelihoods that what one has observed really is significant.

What were the factors that guided the choices made? What apparent connections between dream and name? Here are a few examples. The man stimulated with the name *Jenny*, the name of a previous girl-friend whom he had described as a red-head, dreamed of opening a safe with a *jemmy*. 'The only thing that was in colour was the jemmy . . . a sort of red . . . it seemed to stand out.' After the name *Sheila* had been played, another man reported that he had dreamed he had left behind his book at the University, his copy of *Schiller*, the German poet and philosopher. A girl during whose dream *Robert* had been played, described a dream in which she looked at a film of a *rabbit*, which looked 'distorted'.

In these instances we can see the operation of rhyming, assonant or 'clang' associations. The sound of the word determined the sense of the dream. It was with remarkable insight that, long before such experiments, in the year 1918, Carl Gustav Jung wrote, 'Were we to succeed in producing responses in a sleeping person, clang-responses would certainly be the exclusive results'. Not, in practice, exclusive, but certainly more frequent. We can detect another element in red-headed Jenny eliciting a red-handled jemmy, and Robert the 'distorted' rabbit. It is as if, quietly ruminating on the stimulus, the mind has been tracked off into considerations of the stimulus features and characteristics, how 'Robert' was not quite the right name for a rabbit, how it was somehow distorted. We see these side-tracking associations put into concrete form: the red handle of the jemmy.

The same process is seen in the case of another man to whom *Gillian* was played. This was the name of an ex-girl-friend. Half way through a long dream report he described the entry of an old woman who 'came from Chile'. She was a Chilean (Gillian), an old woman (ex-girl-friend). In the dream she ran about on wet rocky ground with bare feet. Which might have made her feet chilly!

Another purely assonant connection was seen in an example where the sound of the word seemed to have been, as it were, meditated upon by the sleeping mind in a verbally playful way, so that the stimulus, *Naomi*, elicited a dream description which began: 'We were travelling North, having an aim to ski. My friend, he said "Oh?"' If one says these words to oneself one hears the 'clang' at once. '*An aim* to ski' (NAoMI). 'He said, "Oh?"' (NaOmi).

Examples like the last can be found in some of the older medical literature about dream interpretation. Sigmund Freud discussed a dream in which were references to Italy, to (before translation) *gen Italien*, which he took as play upon the word *Genitalien* (genitals). Another excellent example of dream word-play is mentioned in a book written by Dr W. Bonime who uses dream interpretations as talking points with his patients. The woman chemist whose life was being made wretched by the association with her lover, dreamed of being poisoned by cardiac glucosides. The latter is the name of a class of drugs much used in the treatment of heart failure. Glucose = sweetness, cardiac = heart. Her life was being poisoned through the sweet-heart at her side (cardiac glucoside).

Berger's experiments, though revealing easily identifiable 'clang' ties between name and dream content, revealed also more devious connections. The last were not readily apparent to an external judge like myself, but came to light when, finally, all the volunteers were recalled by day, everything was explained to them, and each listened to his or her own dream tape-recordings, and guessed which name must have accompanied which dream. It could be argued that theirs were not unbiased judgements, as mine perforce had to be, for it could be claimed that some subconscious memory of the name persisted in their minds in association with each dream. As might be expected, they scored rather more correct hits than I had, for they had information I did not possess. One girl had described a dream involving a dress shop. Where I could see no obvious connection she at once chose correctly the stimulus that had been used, namely *Richard*, the name of an Edinburgh fashion shop of which she had been a customer shortly before the experiments.

An example where the connection was more disguised was that where the girl, a local girl, had an Indian boy-friend, called Leslie. Racial prejudice unhappily being what it is, even in a cosmopolitan city such as Edinburgh with many students from overseas, the relationship was a source of some emotional conflict for her family and herself. In her dream, containing a great deal of sexual symbolism (of which more later), she mentioned an Indian woman who wore glasses. The stimulus had been *Leslie*. An Indian woman would not be a source of emotional conflict or anxiety. Leslie, who wore glasses, had he figured in this sex-bound dream, might well have been. Apparent disguising of dream content, as if to prevent anxiety-provoking stuff, was the subject of much comment by Freud. He regarded dreams as guardians of sleep, as means whereby our earthy urges are allowed some expression in disguised form, lacking which disguise they might so shock our tender consciences that we should waken in a state of alarm.

In this connection it is interesting that the laboratory setting should now be known to exert a decent restraining influence on earthy urges during dreams. Thin gauges fixed to the eyelids can be used to wake a person at home from rapid eye movement periods so that he can at once record his dream. Comparison between large numbers of dream reports American citizens have made at home and those they have made in laboratories show that, in their content, home dreams are definitely spicier! I do not really believe we can attribute the extra spiciness to more television-viewing at home but in New York experimenters showed movie films to twelve men just before bed-time and made very interesting findings. Six men saw on their first night a horrifying film of an Australian aboriginal initiation rite involving a surgical operation on the penis carried out with the aid of a sharp stone and a hot fire, while six saw only a pleasant travel film. The next night each got the film he had not previously seen.

The experience of what the authors, without hyperbole, called the 'stress' film was followed by sleep with rapid eye movements in greater profusion and with more frequent awakenings from the rapid eye movement periods. It could be inferred that the stress film left the mind and brain in a greater degree of turmoil, that the dreams were more vivid, and that they were more likely to lead to awakenings. Parents of television-viewing children take note!

Symbolism

The Indian woman in the dream could be interpreted as Leslie in disguise. She represented him. She symbolized him. In the other dreams *gen Italien* was a symbol for genitals, 'cardiac glucoside' for sweetheart. In the waking state our brains function efficiently, we display a precise and discriminative wit. In drowsiness, as we saw in Chapter 2, and in dreams, the precision is lost, the barriers between one idea and another become less defined, what they have in common flows together and the dreamer does not sharply discriminate between them. The one becomes the equal of the other. The one can symbolize the other. Some people believe this symbolization in dreams is a very subtle affair, that it is always done 'on purpose'. At all events, symbolization in dreams is common, and has long been recognized as such. Former generations regarded dreams as prophetic, as omens or guides, and venerated those who interpreted dreams. In the Book of Genesis, we read how Joseph, the boy with the coat of many colours, infuriated his elder brothers with his stories of his dreams:

And Joseph dreamed a dream. . . . For, behold we were binding sheaves in the field, and lo, my sheaf arose, and also stood upright; and, behold, your sheaves stood round about, and made obeisance to my sheaf.

And his brethren said to him, 'Shalt thou indeed reign over us? Or shalt thou indeed have dominion over us?' And they hated him yet the more for his dreams. . . .

And Joseph went after his brethren, and found them in Dothan . . . they said one to another, Behold, this dreamer cometh . . . let us slay him . . . and we shall see what will become of his dreams . . . and Judah said . . ., let us sell him to the Ishmaelites . . . into Egypt. . . .

And Pharaoh said unto Joseph, I have dreamed a dream, and there is none can interpret it. . . . And Joseph said unto Pharaoh, The dream of Pharaoh is one: God hath shewed Pharaoh what he is about to do. The seven good kine are seven years and the seven good ears are seven years: the dream is one. . . . And let them gather all the food of those good years that come, and lay up corn . . . against the seven years of famine. . . .

And Pharaoh said unto Joseph, See, I have set thee over all the land of Egypt. . . .

Sigmund Freud rejected the prophetic role of dreams. He retained another of the ancient notions, that certain symbols always have a specific meaning for all men. Thus, for Freud's followers, who are called psycho-analysts, if three men all mention an apple in their dreams, each is speaking symbolically of a breast. In the U.S.A., Calvin Hall has objected to this universal application of dream interpretation. He has argued cogently (and for me convincingly) that the meaning of a dream symbol depends upon the personality and background of the individual person. A dream of a cow might symbolize the nourishing mother for one man; for another, who feared such animals in waking life, a cow in a dream might symbolize his fears.

An assumption of psycho-analytic theory is that our every thought or action has a purpose in maintaining emotional and bodily equilibrium, and, in particular, that dreams are all wish-fulfilling. Lots of us have day-dreams – of making advances to some pretty girl we know, or of wearing a mink coat while driving to a theatre first night – which could certainly be said to be wish-fulfilling. Getting what we should like in a world of make-believe. But are all dreams like that? Are all the crazy concoctions of drowsiness really important? Are not many of them simply the aimless meanderings of a mechanism which is only just managing to tick over? That everything must be determined, or explicable, in terms of the interaction of different forces, was integral in Freud's thinking, the thinking of a late-nineteenth-century man. In that century, mechanics and predictable mechanisms were conquering the world. Only in the twentieth century did physics advance to the acceptance that not all physical events were predictable or determined, that some were subject to indeterminism.

The belief that dreams are wish-fulfilling has been examined at times by questioning very hungry or very thirsty men about their dreams, but Freud's claim that hungry men dreamed of feasts, or thirsty men of drink was not confirmed. This failure of confirmation does not impress analysts, who regard the manifest content of dreams (what the individual describes) as unimportant and simply a cloak for the so-called latent content (hidden meanings). In the latent content, hidden in the Unconscious, the wish-fulfilment would be manifest. Unfortunately, no one can examine the Unconscious except through inference.

Psycho-analysts believe that reprehensible thoughts, words and deeds are kept out of our waking behaviour by a process called repression, that in fact there is always a form of censorship operating, even when we are alone, at the command of our super-ego or conscience. The censorship is less strongly exercised upon our fantasy life, especially our dreams, though even there the latent content, the earthy urges, are disguised into relative respectability in the manifest content. We forget dreams, so it is supposed, because of a further act of censorship during waking hours. The scientific investigator of dreaming would reply that the latter assumption of censorship is unnecessary, that extent of recall depends upon the strength of the memory traces initially formed, and that when the cerebral cortex is not working with optimum efficiency, sufficiently strong memory traces are not formed. The failure to recall dreams does not require the assumption of a prudish censor any more than failure of recall after drunkenness or severe head injury, in which two circumstances also the cerebral cortex is not able to work at its best.

In an experimental study of twenty American men who were wakened from their dreams during the night and then, to their surprise, asked to recall the dreams again in the morning, the dream memories were poor. Over a third were completely forgotten in the morning. Whether or not a dream was remembered was found to be governed by the profusion of rapid eye movements (which, as we have seen, relates to dream vividness), by the speediness with which the volunteer woke up and gave his answer during the night, and on whether he was awake for long.

The more quickly he had dropped off to sleep again, the less he remembered in the morning. A psycho-analyst, who had studied the night dream reports, and the volunteers' personalities, and had made predictions about which dreams would have been repressed by the morning, was not successful.

Sex Dreams

In the next chapter we shall see that sleep with rapid eye movements is a special kind of sleep with characteristic bodily accompaniments. It is a kind of sleep which, because it occupies a lot of the sleeping time in the newborn, and because of the parts of the brain which govern it, has been called primitive or archaic sleep. The regions of the brain which control it are the power-houses for other primitive forms of behaviour, including emotional expression and mating activity. There seems to be some overlap, or special connection of function, between the dreaming sleep and sexual activity. Female rabbits after copulation rapidly pass into that kind of sleep, which is then interrupted by snuffling and licking around the perineum. In a number of sleep-research laboratories it has been shown that, in the human male, erections of the penis accompany rapid eye movement periods.

Many an ordinary citizen tends to equate psychology with the study of sex, a mistake attributable to the emphasis placed by Sigmund Freud upon the sexual drive, following his experience with a number of middle-European young women patients of the late nineteenth century. He took the view that much dream content illustrates sexual themes. An interesting survey was carried out by Dr Calvin Hall, who, reading through psycho-analytic books and articles, made lists of the commonly occurring dream objects or activities which psycho-analysts took to be symbolic of sexual organs or activities. Thus he found 102 dream symbols for penis, such as stick, gun or pen, and fifty-five symbols for coitus, such as to ride, to shoot, to plough or to thrash, flog or belt.

You might argue that this list simply showed that psycho-analysts were a bunch of dirty-minded men who would twist sex out of anything. But Calvin Hall then went through Partridge's

Dictionary of Slang and Unconventional English and noted down all the slang words, or coarse expressions, for sexual organs and activities. There were 200 for penis, including stick, gun and horn, and 212 for coitus, including flog, belt, thrash and screw.

Many of these coarse expressions had been in the English language for centuries. So there were dirty-minded Englishmen before there were dirty-minded psycho-analysts. But are these representations characteristic only of lewd men? Or do they shine through even the dreams of average, delicately-nurtured citizens? The psycho-analytic data suggests that they do, and, for my own part, I would be inclined to accept that they do. Let us take some examples.

Sexual symbolism is common in waking life. Few healthy men could claim to pass without a glance a window display of foundation-garments, as they are called. More extreme are so-called fetishists for whom such diverse objects as black and shiny boots, black and shiny leather clothing, plastic bags (potentially dangerous, these), rubber coats, handbags, or per-ambulators are favoured as necessary adjuncts to sexual excite-ment. Many fetishistic activities are clearly symbolic. Recently, in the newspapers there was an account of the wife who divorced her husband because he made her wear a rubber mackintosh and stand in the garden or the bath while he sprayed her with a hose-pipe. Another young man went round chemists' shops seeking a pretty girl from whom to purchase, and who would hand to him, a baby's dummy or teat. Another variant is the gentleman who presses the glowing tip of his cigarette upon the lady's dress and burns a hole into it.

Bearing in mind this last example of day-time symbolism, consider the following two dreams. The first description was of a recurrent type of dream, described by a respectable middle-class Edinburgh woman of sixty-four years during her first psychiatric interview, and reiterated for verbatim recording during her second interview. Some of the latter follows.

PATIENT: Of course my father used to thrash me a lot. He was very strict and religious.

DOCTOR: He beat you, did he?

PATIENT: Mmmhm. One of those long, stinging canes that they used to have in the old days. Like a walking-stick but bamboo. Any time I did anything wrong. He even used to sit with one on the table at me when I was eating my food. . . .

[*She grew up to be afraid of a man who would thrash her with his stick.*]

PATIENT: And I have bad dreams, some of being imprisoned, someone after me, somebody always after me, or somebody won't let me go . . . last week . . . I was captured, and a man put a lighted cigar down my, down here.

DOCTOR: Down where?

PATIENT: Down my blouse, and I pulled it out again.

DOCTOR: And then what happened?

PATIENT: He stuck a cigarette on the end of my, my cheek.

DOCTOR: And that was lighted too?

PATIENT: Uhha.

DOCTOR: You could see the red end, could you?

PATIENT: Uhha.

[The expression 'Uhha' is a local dialect word commonly used as a substitute for 'Yes'. Notice that she said the 'end of my', then hesitated before 'cheek'. 'End of' would not normally be applied to the word 'cheek'. Many people speak of the buttocks as having two cheeks.]

DOCTOR: You get on with your husband all right?

PATIENT: Uhha. We have to, after forty-two years! Well, you sort of get into the pattern of each other. Oh, we get on all right.

DOCTOR: You get on all right? Last time, you said, I think, that it wasn't sort of romantic –

PATIENT: No.

DOCTOR: What was it you said? If you ever got another husband –

PATIENT: Oh, are you going to bring that all up! I said he would need to be physically handicapped!

DOCTOR: You wouldn't want –

PATIENT: Oh, my goodness, no.

Leaving this representative of an older generation, terrified of a man with a stick, a man with a glowing cigar or cigarette, let us now consider another dream, told in the same year, 1962, by a girl university student of twenty-one, when Berger awoke her from a rapid eye movement period. The only child of rather old parents, she had had a boy-friend briefly when aged seventeen, and now had the Indian boy-friend mentioned on page 83.

Consider too the circumstances. When one seeks volunteers for scientific experiments one does so in a brisk, cold manner by a written circular. But what, in reality, is the situation? In effect, a good-looking and charming young man, Ralph Berger, makes overtures – 'Will you come and sleep . . . with me? . . . I want to do some experiments.' She hesitates, then agrees. (Only under pressure from me was Ralph Berger persuaded to allow me to portray the situation in this way!)

She goes alone one night to meet Berger. In the bedroom she dons her night attire, emerges and enters the EEG room where she is given close personal attention. Little silver tokens are planted upon the skin of her face, her hair is gently parted and further tokens affixed. They go together to the bedroom, she climbs into bed, he attaches the wires from her head to a box above her so that she is now tied to the bed. Having, if only figuratively, tucked her up, he puts out the light and bids her sleep, saying that he will disturb her later in the night. On this, her first night, you might suppose she would lie there awhile, thinking, 'What next? . . . will he, might he re-enter and . . . and if he did, well, no, but, well, if, but, no, perhaps . . . .'

She took several hours to fall asleep, so that there was only one rapid eye movement period that night. She was awakened from it. She described how she 'had been tossing and turning', but finally had slept and dreamed that Berger did come into the room. 'You were dressed in a top hat, morning suit, and you were smoking a cigar. And someone handed me a cigarette which had been lit at the tipped end and at the other end [pause]. And I smoked it [pitch of voice rising], but I wasn't burned or anything.' Berger then inquired, 'You smoked it? How did you smoke it?' She replied, 'At the tipped end. Normally – [pause]. It was all sort of frayed and burnt. But I don't know if it was still burning at the end that I smoked it.' Berger – 'I see, you sucked on the burnt end?' 'Yes, and I remember I inhaled [giggle, giggle], because I don't normally inhale.'

We see once more the glowing cigar and cigarette. The girl who did not normally inhale (giggle, giggle). But this time she did. Berger entered the room wearing a morning suit: tails. It was not he who handed her the cigarette. Just as (p. 83) she evaded Leslie in her dream, so here also she side-stepped, she did not, directly from Berger, accept that which she 'inhaled'.

Let me hasten to acknowledge that these are selected dreams. Not all dreams are like these, and, in my own view, it is only a minority which contain sexual symbolism. The special physiological conditions of the dream state do nevertheless seem to favour sexual themes. While healthy males in the waking state may day-dream along sexual themes, in the absence of concurrent physical stimulation these do not generally lead to a sexual climax or orgasm. In the sleep of male adolescents, however, such dreams, with ejaculation of semen, are both normal and common ('wet dreams'). One such dream, by a young man, was, by chance, recorded in the sleep-laboratory at Edinburgh and occurred during a rapid eye movement period, and another in the laboratory of Dr Charles Fisher in New York.

Fisher studied a series of fifty-eight dreams and made predictions of those in which there would have been sudden change in the degree of penile erection and found he could do so successfully. He correctly predicted seven of the eight instances of sudden loss of erection and five out of six instances of sudden increase. A dream of the second kind was one in which a young man dreamed he was alone in his house looking out of the window. There was a crowd in front of the house. Two girls came and told him a friend of his had committed suicide and then he was unhappy. They came in and he began to tease them. One girl dropped something, a hairpin. He picked it up and gave it to her and held her hand – at this moment he had an ejaculation of semen.

Erections are present in almost all rapid eye movement periods, even though the man be elderly and even though he had sexual intercourse with ejaculation just before sleep. Fisher's study confirmed other laboratory work indicating that the degree of tumescence is smaller during those dreams which an independent judge will consider anxious in nature.

Calvin Hall has collected dream accounts (recalled by day) numbering tens of thousands. Among this collection are many wet dreams, generally of a clearly sexual nature, but also sometimes purely symbolic. Seminal emission accompanied such dream events as climbing stairs or ladders, or car-driving ('the transports of love'). Hall takes issue with the Freudian contention that such symbols are, in a sense, deliberate disguises. The same person one night will have frankly sexual dreams, and on other nights, symbolic dreams. Hall argues convincingly that if the symbolism were there in order to appease the prudish Censor of the psycho-analysts, it should be a consistent and not an occasional feature of such dreams. Symbolic thought is not necessarily or always deliberately disguised thought.

Women too have sexual dreams. When inexperienced, dreams are essentially 'romantic'. Kinsey and his fellow American research workers, who questioned many thousands of women, state that occasional dreams to the point of orgasm occur in a considerable proportion of mature females. Such dreams increase sharply in frequency when other normal outlets are denied them, as when women enter prison, or are separated from their husbands. The tendency towards sexual activity is controlled by chemicals, called hormones, which circulate in the bloodstream and act upon centres in the brain. The urge towards such activity is, therefore, largely of internal origin. Men whose spinal cords have been shattered through injury, so that there is no longer any nervous connection between their brains and their lower bodies, still have sexual dreams in which they experience all the feelings and sensations of orgasm. The basis of this experience is not in their isolated lower bodies. It is wholly within their brains. We cannot ask animals what they have been dreaming about, but dogs, like human males, show erections of the penis from time to time during sleep. The same is true of male shrews (they look like mice with long snouts) in whom pelvic thrusting movements follow the erections and precede awakening. Sleeping bitches, while in heat, sometimes look as if they are dreaming of mating and show episodes of genital engorgement, secretion, pelvic thrusting movements and squealing.

Living in Dreams

Other, less pleasant, features of waking life also can intrude upon the dream-world. Some American psychiatrists collected (by day) twenty dream reports each from six patients who were very depressed. For comparison purposes they collected the same number of dreams from six other people, similar in age and social background to the patients, but who were not suffering from depression. They put code numbers on all the dream reports, mixed them up and gave them to an independent judge to study. He was asked to score each dream in terms of various 'masochistic' features (or self-punishing features, characteristic of daytime thinking when depressed). When eventually the code was broken, it was found that he had noticed far more 'masochistic' features in the dreams of the depressed patients than in the dreams of the other group, the difference being too great to attribute to chance. Themes of rejection and failure were common. 'I was waiting for my friends all night, but they never showed up', or 'My fiancé married somebody else', or 'I ran to make an appointment with you. I was one minute late and the door was locked.'

The most vivid living-in-a-dream is seen, when, after some terrifying event, it is all gone through again and again in dreams. I knew a bus driver who once, through no fault of his own, ran over and killed a little girl. For nights his sleep was disturbed by dreams in which again he cried out and slammed his foot upon the brake, doing so with such force that he broke the wooden bed-end. There are many wartime descriptions of men, recently engaged in combat, who would, by night, dream that they were again in action. They would shout in their sleep, hurl themselves about, rise from their beds, shout orders (using the same phrases night after night), and attack imaginary enemies. The noise of a passing aeroplane or a bang would provoke a state of terror. Some were violent and injured themselves by striking furniture or windows. When spoken to they would reply only with incoherent mumbling, apparently related to battle experiences. Fifteen years after the last war six hundred survivors of Nazi concentration camps were located by L. Eitinger in Norway and Israel. In many survivors there remained a legacy of recurrent nightmares 'with S.S. guards who persecute, hit and shoot, with "selections" where the individual waits endlessly to be chosen and sent to his death, where the tension seems unbearable and where the patients are woken by their own screams or by their mates'.'

There are cases recorded in both English and American law where it has been held that a homicidal act during the night was committed during sleep and the person charged has been acquitted of murder.

Sleep-walking as an occasional event is normal for most children. There is a strong tendency for it to run in families. Among some children it is an indication of emotional disturbance. The child may walk about with a blank expression, mumbling to himself. He may fumble with objects, and bump into things but generally avoids major obstacles. He may appear distressed and preoccupied. Attempts to waken him meet only very gradually with success. Left to himself he will return to bed after some minutes. In the morning there is complete lack of memory for the events of the night. Occasionally he may have injured himself and the sleep-walking is not without danger through a liability to falls from windows or down stairs.

Research in Los Angeles has shown that sleep-walking episodes never occur during rapid eye movement periods. They arise mainly in the first hours of sleep and exclusively in sleep with large slow EEG waves. EEG sleep rhythms continue to some degree throughout the walking period. The old idea of sleep-walking enacting a dream has found little support. The walking does not arise from rapid eye movement periods in which the majority of elaborate dreams seem to occur. In so far as the walking betrays an unquiet mind it may confirm the presence of mental life in orthodox sleep (see p. 70).

5. Two Kinds of Sleep

The recurring periods of rapid eye movements during a normal night's sleep are accompanied by an EEG very similar to that of drowsiness. Furthermore, the periods are accompanied by an elevation in the degree of consciousness, a consciousness not of the outside world, but of an inwardly-created, dream world. The Chicago pioneers understandably extended traditional ideas about the depth of sleep to the recurrent changes that they saw each night, and proposed that the rapid eye movement periods were periods of light sleep, that sleep became light about once every one and a half hours. Their work stimulated research throughout the world into the cyclical pattern of sleep, and gradually it emerged that it was not so much a matter of change in sleep depth, as of alternation between two very different kinds of sleep.

Dr Bill Dement moved on from human volunteers to cats, and found that, in their sleep too, there were rapid eye movement periods accompanying a low voltage EEG (which in the cat looks more like that of wakefulness than drowsiness, although carefully analysis of the rhythm frequencies show them to be slower than those of wakefulness). At these times the cat twitched his whiskers and flicked his tail and an onlooker might have said, 'That cat's dreaming!'

At Lyons in France, Dr Michel Jouvet began a brilliant analysis of this sleep of cats. He noticed that when the cat passed into sleep with high voltage EEG slow waves and motionless eyes, the cat, lying on its tummy with paws tucked in front of its chest, still held its head up slightly. When a rapid eye movement period began, the cat's head flopped down. He made electrical records of muscle activity simultaneously with those of the EEG and eye movements. Always in sleep with big slow EEG waves the muscles at the back of the neck remained tense, but they relaxed totally whenever the sleep with low voltage EEG and rapid eye movements began.

If the latter kind of sleep was 'light' sleep in man, obviously it was not in the cat, whose muscles were then most relaxed. Fine wires were implanted into the reticular formation of a cat and electrical stimulation applied to awaken it from sleep (see p. 26). A far stronger stimulus was needed during the rapid eye movement period than during sleep with big, slow EEG waves and tense muscles. So research workers studying cats began to call the sleep with rapid eye movements 'deep sleep' at the same time as those who studied humans were calling it 'light sleep'. Jouvet continued on his way. He made carefully localized zones of damage within the brain-stem of cats. If he damaged the central reticular formation then, as expected, perpetual sleep resulted. But not with *continuous* big slow EEG waves. Although an outside noise could no longer cause low voltage fast EEG waves to appear in the cerebral cortex, if he just waited, then, from time to time, for periods of several minutes, the EEG would change to a low voltage one and the neck muscles would go slack. If he made localized damage in the brain-stem less centrally, he found places where, despite the damage, ordinary awakening was still possible, yet the cerebral cortex no longer showed low voltage fast EEG waves periodically during sleep although the muscles nevertheless went slack at certain times. It looked as if he were interrupting an ascending pathway from some lower centre which could send up impulses to change the cortical EEG pattern. He found a region in the lower part of the brain, in the part of the 'hind-brain' called the pons, which seemed to act as a controlling centre for what other workers were calling 'deep' sleep of cats. Electrical stimulation there can quickly bring on this phase of sleep and make it last longer. So Jouvet called it the 'hind-brain phase' or 'paradoxical phase' of sleep. Jouvet tried recording the muscle tension from the back of the neck in humans too. Would they in their 'light' sleep with rapid eye movements show a paradoxical loss of muscle tension? They relaxed so much as soon as they passed into sleep that it was impossible to say. There was no scope for further relaxation.

At Edinburgh we were looking to see if, when there were rapid eye movements in dreams, the muscles around the larynx, or voice-box, would also show sudden activity that might mean silent dream-talking. My colleague, Ralph Berger, noticed how the muscles round the larynx always relaxed much more as soon as a rapid eye movement period began. If the human, too, relaxed much more during rapid eye movement periods, then, we realized, we should have to stop calling it 'light sleep'.

Actually, the throat muscle relaxation is the first sign that a rapid eye movement period is starting, and though it is rather a bother, on technical grounds, it is nowadays often recorded during human sleep in laboratories all over the world.

So we came to call the rapid eye movement periods 'paradoxical sleep' in humans too. And if we used that name, then 'orthodox' sleep was an appropriate name for the other kind of sleep, which had been studied quite a lot in the past. Paradoxical sleep is often called REM (frequently pronounced 'rem' to rhyme with gem) sleep, as an abbreviation of rapid eye movement sleep. Orthodox sleep is, alas, often called NREM sleep – an unpronounceable combination of letters – for non-rapid eye movement sleep (frequently in speaking called 'non-rem', again rhyming with gem). Figure 7 illustrates the two kinds of sleep. They have in their time had many names and there is still no final agreement. To my mind REM sleep is an inappropriate name. Moles, for example, spend a quarter of their sleeping hours in paradoxical sleep. They are blind, have only rudimentary eyeball muscles, and have no rapid eye movements, so it would seem nonsensical if I were to have just written that they spend a quarter of the time in rapid eye movement or REM sleep. Incidentally the fact that moles get such a lot of paradoxical sleep shows that it serves a more fundamental purpose than just keeping the eyeballs exercised in readiness for waking use – a seriously discussed contemporary hypothesis.

We continue breathing throughout sleep, so not all the muscles of the body are paralysed during paradoxical sleep. But most are, even to the extent of abolition of the normal reflex twitch of the leg muscles, which in the waking state, and in orthodox sleep, follows involuntarily upon sudden stimulation of a nerve carry-

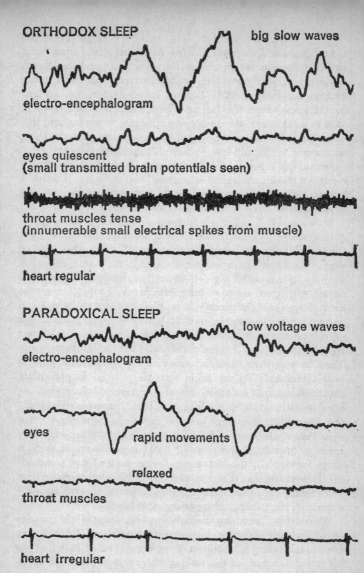

ORTHODOX SLEEP

big slow waves

electro-encephalogram

eyes quiescent
(small transmitted brain potentials seen)

throat muscles tense
(innumerable small electrical spikes from muscle)

heart regular

PARADOXICAL SLEEP

low voltage waves

electro-encephalogram

eyes   rapid movements

relaxed

throat muscles

heart irregular

Fig 7. The characteristics of the two kinds of sleep.

ing messages from sense organs to the spinal cord. Although the cat's body flops, its whiskers may twitch, and lots of little facial twitches accompany human rapid eye movements, while the chimpanzee's face is grotesquely distorted by ceaseless grimacing. What is more, the paralysis is momentarily, but quite frequently, interrupted by sudden movements of a limb or some other large part of the body; indeed it has been claimed that, on average, the part of the body which moves is related to some dream action; that the right arm moves slightly when a right-handed person dreams of throwing a stone. Nerve impulses descend down the spinal cord to cause the paralysis and stop the nerve cells there from firing off messages which could bring muscles into action. These descending impulses are suddenly intensified with each burst of rapid eye movements. The twitches of the limbs usually accompany a burst of rapid eye movements, so it looks as if there are special precautions to stop us moving our arm just at the very moment of dreaming of throwing a stone!

The twitches and sudden eye movements are classed among *phasic* components of paradoxical sleep, whereas the *tonic* or more persistent features include the rather low-voltage EEG, the muscle flaccidity and the erections of the penis. Other phasic features much studied in animals include 'PGO spikes' or ponto-geniculo-occipital spikes, indicating the parts of the brain where high voltage electrical discharges suddenly occur in bursts, often roughly associated in time with the rapid eye movements. The PGO spikes are more central in the brain but should not be thought of as therefore in some way more fundamental or important: they themselves are preceded by another phasic event, namely change of heart rate, which is itself governed by nervous impulses from the brain.

Major body movements, on a number-per-minute basis, were twice as frequent during paradoxical sleep as during orthodox sleep, in a group of middle-aged Edinburgh citizens. The greater restlessness during that kind of sleep would once have been seen as a reason to call it 'light' sleep. In the cat the electrical firing of the cells of the cerebral cortex is much reduced in orthodox sleep compared with wakefulness. In paradoxical sleep, on the other hand, the firing rates are about the same as in wakefulness, but the rhythmic patterns of firing are quite different and less well organized. It might have been tempting to call paradoxical sleep 'light' sleep because of the similarity to wakefulness in cell firing rate, but the patterning emphasizes that we should do better to think of it as different in kind rather than degree.

The facial twitchings in man occur very strikingly during nightmare dreams. This is a topic upon which new light has been cast by studies of paradoxical sleep, because past writers about nightmares have defined them not only as unpleasant dreams but ones in which the dreamer feels unable to move. Borne helplessly towards some hideous fate the terrified dreamer struggles to escape, but finds himself paralysed, his body seemingly divorced from his conscious efforts. As he struggles, intermittent twitches and strangled cries interrupt the bursts of rapid eye movement and the paradoxical sleep EEG record, till, after half a minute, he finally wakes. Our new knowledge enables us to understand that he really was paralysed.

There are other short nightmare-type experiences divorced from any lengthy or complex dream and from which there may be sudden awakening with a sense of intense fear. Like sleepwalking these episodes occur in orthodox sleep. In children they are called night-terrors, and are particularly distressing for the parents who try to comfort their suddenly screaming child, who himself remembers nothing of the incident in the morning even though he sat up staring and whimpering for several minutes. Night-terrors are occasionally experienced in adults too. Early in the night there is an abrupt arousal from orthodox sleep with the very largest and slowest of EEG waves (called Stage 4). Groans or terrible shrieks accompany sudden clambering out of bed, with rapid and deep breathing and a pounding of the heart up to 160 beats per minute. Immediate questioning will often elicit a single, brief, frightening thought, or image, such as an intruder in the room, but otherwise all is forgotten and only the family may retain an unforgettable memory.

The experience of wanting desperately to escape from a dream, but being paralysed, is especially common in a disorder known as narcolepsy. Patients with this disorder are abnormally liable to fall asleep. Especially when bored, or under conditions of monotony, when on buses or trains (or, a serious matter in the Services, when on guard duty) or when rhythmically walking (they bump into people and appear drunk – very embarrassing), or chewing their food. The last tendency to fall asleep over the dessert is especially amusing to their friends, but not to the patients themselves. A unique feature of their disorder is that, when they fall asleep, after a minute of ordinary drowsiness, they often pass at once into paradoxical sleep (whereas normally people always pass into orthodox sleep). Having gained, as it were, their ration of, say, fifteen minutes paradoxical sleep, they may awaken, and then, when dropping off again a few minutes later, always pass into orthodox sleep, as if the primary need (see p. 102) for paradoxical sleep had been satisfied. The passage direct into paradoxical sleep now explains why it has, for many years, been well known that these people have vivid dream experiences during their naps.

Quite often these narcoleptic patients (and normal people less often) describe 'sleep paralysis'. It is rather doubtful whether there is any real difference between this and a nightmare, for it consists of an unpleasant dream in which there is a vague awareness of being, for instance, in one's own bedroom, yet feeling or seeing headless monsters or threatening enemies in the room, coupled with a desire to move but a paralysis of the body.

Another characteristic complaint of these patients is of 'cataleptic' attacks. These are sudden attacks of paralysis lasting a few seconds during the day. The individual may crumple and fall to the floor, or just the jaw and arms may sag for a couple of seconds. Always they are provoked by a sudden emotion. Laughter, anger or fear are most common. Everyday expressions like 'helpless with laughter', 'speechless with anger' and 'paralysed with fear' suggest that to some degree the same mechanisms may be operative in all of us.

A narcoleptic patient of mine has for years now crumpled up whenever she laughs heartily. If she has a funny story to tell, she always sits down first! Another, a man, gets his attacks whenever he suddenly feels a surge of triumph. 'When I've outsmarted someone.' Two male patients have both told me how, when moved to sudden anger by their adolescent sons, upon raising a hand to cuff the youths, they would suddenly collapse into paralysis. The best story is that of the woman who dearly loved a game of cards, but, whenever she got a really good hand and felt a thrill of excitement, her jaw would sag involuntarily so that her secret was betrayed. It seems probable that, at the moment of paralysis, the nervous system of these patients is momentarily in a state resembling that of paradoxical sleep, during which also they are paralysed. It will be remembered (see p. 87) that the zones within the brain regulating emotion overlap in function with those controlling paradoxical sleep.

The group of mammals known as ruminants – cows, sheep, goats and others – go on 'ruminating', or cud-chewing, throughout the night. They go on doing this while asleep, even though their eyes remain open. (After all, we keep our ears open and our digestive functions also continue during sleep.) They become unresponsive to things going on around them and have the EEG of sleep. The peculiar arrangement of their upper digestive tract relies upon gravity for its proper function. In consequence the head and neck have to remain erect even during sleep. What, we may ask, will happen if their muscles become paralysed during paradoxical sleep so that they cannot keep up their heads. Will their food 'go the wrong way'?

They get round this little problem by eschewing paradoxical sleep. The lamb before weaning spends much of the night in paradoxical sleep. As he grows older and begins to ruminate, paradoxical sleep is almost lost. Only rarely does it briefly appear, and at these times rumination ceases. This is very interesting: it implies that his brain processes have matured in such a fashion that they need scarcely any of the particular restitutive virtues which one must assume normally stem from paradoxical sleep.

The Need for Paradoxical Sleep

When six Edinburgh medical students had been kept awake for 108 hours and were then allowed to sleep, on the first night they spent most of the night in orthodox sleep, and spent far less than normal in paradoxical sleep. They had been very sleepy people.

Did they therefore take an excess of orthodox sleep because it was 'deeper' sleep?

When six women who were drug addicts and had for years taken large quantities of amphetamine-containing pills (the so-called 'purple-hearts' and similar preparations) were suddenly deprived of their customary source of pep, their nervous systems were so unaccustomed to the situation that the ladies had difficulty in keeping awake. They were very sleepy people. Would they, like the sleep-deprived sleepy people, take more orthodox sleep? No. When they slept, they spent twice as much as normal of the night in paradoxical sleep, as if, for them, that was the 'deeper' sleep: one more good reason for concluding that we must no longer talk about one or other of the two kinds of sleep being 'deeper'.

We do not know why we sleep, we just know we have got to. If there are two kinds of sleep, one would expect each to be needed. When those sleep-deprived Edinburgh students had given first priority to an excess of orthodox sleep on their first recovery night, the next night, they spent an abnormal excess of the night in paradoxical sleep, as if catching up on what they had not got the previous night. This was an observation which served to confirm some important experiments carried out by Dr Bill Dement, who, by that time, had moved his work to New York.

Dement had noticed that when he had kept wakening a volunteer from his dreams, the next night it seemed that rapid eye movement periods began more often than normal. Could it be, thought Dement, that when people were awakened and prevented from continuing a dream, that they were deprived of something important? Could it be that the next night they were attempting to catch up? There was only one way to find out. To do an experiment. A very arduous one.

Watching the electrical tracings throughout night after night, Dement deliberately awakened his volunteers from sleep whenever he was sure a rapid eye movement period had just begun. Normal people, it will be recalled, always pass into orthodox sleep when they fall asleep. This meant that when one of Dement's volunteers had been prevented from getting, say, the normal twenty-minute stretch of paradoxical sleep, and had been limited to a mere three or four minutes before he was awakened for a few minutes, he then always fell once more into orthodox sleep. Over the whole night he would, consequently, become selectively deprived of paradoxical or dreaming sleep. It seemed, however, as if the nervous system imperiously demanded paradoxical sleep, as if the deprivation caused a build-up of 'pressure', for, as the night passed, paradoxical sleep appeared more and more often, until thirty or more awakenings each night were necessary to try and prevent it. Then, finally, an undisturbed night of sleep was allowed. Compared with nights of normal sleep which had been recorded for comparison purposes at the outset of the experiment, the night of undisturbed sleep after deprivation included an excessively large proportion of paradoxical sleep. When results for all the volunteers were pooled, the excess was shown by statistical calculation to be greater than could reasonably be attributed to chance variation. (As with all biological functions, variations from night to night must be expected in any individual.)

As a check Dement got his volunteers to return some weeks later. Again he woke them repeatedly in the night. This time, instead of waking them from rapid eye movement periods, he woke them from orthodox sleep. It was important to find out if the mere fact of repeated awakenings lay at the root of what he had observed. But the awakenings from orthodox sleep did not have the effect that the earlier awakenings had had. Therefore, Dement concluded, the awakenings from the rapid eye movement periods had deprived the individual of something he really needed. At that time Dement was working in a department headed by an unusually experimentally-minded psycho-analyst, Dr Charles Fisher. Consistent with the milieu in which he then worked, Dement proposed that there must exist a 'need to dream' and that his experiments were 'dream-deprivation' experiments. At that time, 1960, the realization that the sleep with rapid eye movements was a physiologically distinct kind of sleep had not really dawned upon sleep researchers.

In more recent times Dement has re-formulated his views and there is now fairly general agreement that we should speak of a need for paradoxical sleep, rather than a need to dream. You might argue that to speak of a need to dream and of a need for paradoxical sleep are equally valid alternatives, the one a formulation in psychological terms, the other a formulation in bodily or physiological terms. But if one theoretical formulation cannot take cognisance of half the data, whereas the other can, then the latter must be preferred.

We now know drugs which will, without any prior 'dream-deprivation', cause an increase of paradoxical sleep. Other drugs are known that will eliminate all signs of paradoxical sleep and of its special dream-like features of mental life and which, even if taken for a year, do not cause daytime mental disorder.

A psychological theory of a need to dream cannot handle these particular observations, whereas physiological theories are happy to be associated with pharmacological data. In this case it would be supposed that the chemical balance, underlying the control of paradoxical sleep, had been suddenly interfered with, by changing the patient's drug intake.

The presence of two, alternating kinds of sleep, clearly analogous to what is seen in the human, has now been discovered in numerous other animal species, so that one can reasonably argue that experiments upon cat paradoxical sleep are relevant to human sleep with rapid eye movements. At Lyons, Jouvet made cuts through the brain-stem, separating the lower part wholly from the upper part, or even removing the latter completely, including the cerebral cortex. What might be called the rear-brained cat still went on alternating between two kinds of sleep, as far as could be judged by the appearance and disappearance of muscle tension and other bodily signs. Whenever the muscle tension vanished, as in the paradoxical sleep of the intact animal, a strong electric shock was applied to the leg, muscle tension returned and the animal appeared to be 'awake' for a few minutes. When the cat's sleep was thus repeatedly interrupted the signs of paradoxical sleep returned with greater and greater frequency and, just as Dement's volunteers needed awakening more and more often, so electric shocks were needed more and more often. In fact it was possible to deprive selectively the rear-brained animal of paradoxical sleep. Once again attempts at 'compensation' followed. One could not possibly attribute dreaming to a rear-brained cat, so one could not say this particular form of meat was 'dream-deprived'. Only a physiological interpretation is possible.

The initial experiments in selective deprivation of paradoxical sleep by Dement raised the question whether a 'need to dream' might be associated with psychological peculiarities by day. Some research has suggested that, by night, human paradoxical sleep is made more intense, with more profuse rapid eye movements and more vivid dreams (see p. 77) as a consequence of selective deprivation. Daytime *sequelae*, such as increased sexiness and gluttony, have been seen in cats, and mild personality changes in man, but in man no dramatic psychological consequence can yet be said to have been demonstrated, certainly none that might not be attributed to partial sleep loss of both kinds or to the action of drugs used to assist selective paradoxical sleep deprivation. We should of course remember that sixty years of laboratory research into total sleep deprivation were needed before a test was found which would demonstrate a measurable impairment consequent upon sleep loss. One day someone will presumably discover a test which will be specifically sensitive to paradoxical sleep loss.

Day-time Cycles Too

There is, however, one possibility which might account for failures to demonstrate impairment, and which might help to explain why, when the subsequent 'compensatory' increase of paradoxical sleep occurs, it is always much less than what was lost. Could the benefits of paradoxical sleep be made up during wakefulness?

When the pioneers in Chicago were looking at sleeping babies and saw an hourly periodicity in sleep they observed that not only was rapid eye movement sleep liable to appear hourly but also, if the baby was on a demand-feeding schedule, he would yell for food at some multiple of that hourly cycle. In New York Dr Charles Fisher and a fellow psycho-analyst made notes over periods of six hours or so whenever people engaged spontaneously in oral activities such as eating, drinking and smoking.

They awarded scores to each example of this behaviour – a drink of milk got a high score because to an analyst it indicates satisfaction of a very primitive or basic need. After ten such sessions it appeared that the oral activity was tending to recur every one and a half hours. It will be remembered that, by night, it is at intervals of one and a half hours that paradoxical sleep appears among adults.

Dr Judith Merrington and I repeated the oral activity experiment, taking precautions to ensure that our volunteers were under a quite false impression of the nature of the study. They never guessed we were interested in their oral behaviour. We took turns to sit behind a one-way viewing screen to note down the times when the ten male and female student volunteers ate or drank. Each was alone – there were no inter-student oral opportunities during the boring six-hour sessions. In their room were foods and drinks of specially low-calorie content in order to avoid any timing-pattern inherent in digestion of high calorie foods. After twenty-seven sessions we were able to confirm the New York findings that, in a free, unstructured environment, there are apparently unsuspected urges which mould our daytime behaviour at about ninety-minute intervals. Since that time other workers have found that general, spontaneous bodily restlessness and the rate of spontaneous work similarly changes every ninety minutes, while in people with epileptic brain rhythms the abnormalities wax and wane every ninety minutes.

There is, therefore, a possibility that when we see paradoxical sleep at night, which is, after all, *during* sleep, we are really seeing signs of a cyclical change in the nervous system which goes on endlessly day and night and tries to impose itself every ninety minutes whether the individual is awake or asleep. The idea was in essence advanced many years earlier by Kleitman and is often referred to as the basic rest–activity cycle – ninety minutes in the human adult, fifty minutes in the baby, shorter still in many animals.

Drugs Reduce Paradoxical Sleep

I mentioned just now the use of drugs for selectively reducing paradoxical sleep and on p. 145 indicate how barbiturate drugs may not only reduce the time spent in that kind of sleep but also the profusion of the accompanying eye movements and the vividness of the accompanying dreams.

Quite small doses of a barbiturate or of amphetamine ('dexedrine') will largely suppress paradoxical sleep by night. Hitherto these two drugs had been regarded as having opposite effects on brain function, the one promoting sleep, the other preventing sleep. Provided a person does sleep after amphetamine, suppression of paradoxical sleep can be seen. Alternatively, if a small quantity of amphetamine is given at the same time as a barbiturate sleeping pill, the suppression of paradoxical sleep is much greater than that which the same dose of barbiturate alone can cause.

Here we see an example of how research in some remote area – the study of dreams – can eventually lead towards new insights into the action of chemicals on nervous tissues, drugs previously regarded as opposites now being seen to share some common properties.

When these drugs, or others, such as a drug called tranylcypromine, are given for a few nights and then stopped, a very large increase in paradoxical sleep follows, even bigger than when the deprivation is effected by means of repeated selective awakening. I mention tranylcypromine because it has become unexpectedly famous. It was introduced a few years ago as a 'mono-amine oxidase inhibitor' for the treatment of certain nervous and mental disorders. When patients getting the drug said to their doctors that they now got headaches whenever they ate cheese, not any old cheese, but a ripe Camembert or Gorgonzola, the doctors just sighed inwardly and did their best to reassure these apparently bizarre people. Eventually truth will out. Ripe cheese contains substances called amines, which cannot be destroyed by the body in the normal way when tranylcypromine has been taken, and headache was one result of this.

We do not know why it is so difficult to prevent a sleep-deprived person from falling into orthodox sleep, or a narcoleptic patient from falling into paradoxical sleep. We assume that some internal chemical imbalance is responsible. It is probably an imbalance within the brain itself and not easily showing in the blood stream. Conjoined (Siamese) twins who share their blood can fall asleep at different times. This does not make it certain that a sleep-promoting substance could not possibly be in the blood, because the balance between sleep and wakefulness, as we saw in Chapter I, is controlled by lots of influences, and a chemical in the blood would be only one. It might be sufficient to tip the balance in one twin, but not in the other, if the latter were excited or interested in something special.

Consequently attempts have been made to induce sleep in animals by injecting fluid taken from the bodies of sleepy animals. W. R. Hess had induced sleep by electrically stimulating the thalamus of the brain (p. 39) and in Switzerland Monnier continued the work by sending rabbits to sleep in this way and then refining some of their blood and injecting its constituents into other rabbits – who then fell asleep. The chemical really responsible was not certain but belonged to a class known as low molecular weight peptides. In the U.S.A. another group of workers kept goats without sleep for 72 hours and then found that in their cerebro-spinal fluid (that forms a water-cushion round the brain) was a low molecular weight substance that, when injected into the brains of rats, made the rats sleep more than was the case if the fluid had come from goats which had not been made sleepy. I think all this adds up in favour of some sleep-chemical being present in body fluids.

It is hard not to believe that such chemicals must exist in the brain itself. We have all experienced difficulty in waking up when we are disturbed from sound sleep. Even though our EEG rhythms may make us appear wide awake within seconds, we nevertheless can take minutes to get a grasp of the situation. In fact it has been shown that the responsiveness of the brain, in terms of evoked potentials (p. 28), is much slower to revive after awakenings from orthodox sleep with the largest and slowest EEG waves than from sleep devoid of very large slow waves.

It is as if we cannot quickly dissipate some sleep-chemical from our systems.

The fact that drugs have been found greatly to alter sleep, and the belief that through chemical studies more will be learned of the nature of sleep, means that we shall have to consider these things more fully in Chapter 7.

6. Hypnosis

Shakespeare had a phrase for everything: the ancient Greeks had gods. From the Greeks come the roots of many of our medical words. The word *hypnosis*, spawned by their god, Hypnos, can be encountered in three settings. First, the state induced by a hypnotic or sleep-promoting drug. We may read about 'barbiturate hypnosis', which is really a state of deliberate mild poisoning or intoxication from which an unnatural state of semi-coma has resulted. Secondly, a state of immobility and compliance (or veritable mouldability) passing into sleep, which can be provoked in diverse creatures by diverse means. Thirdly, a trance state in a human brought about by another man or woman, the hypnotist. It is also a state characterized by compliance or suggestibility, but not by sleep.

Three hundred years ago a man called Kircher described an '*experimentum mirabile*'. Many a farmer's wife must have made the observation long before. When Kircher seized a chicken and held the head and body motionless, while drawing a chalk line outwards from the beak, the chicken became entranced. For some minutes it remained motionless and stupefied. It would also retain any new and unnatural posture imposed upon it. Actually the chalk line is quite unnecessary.

In the last sixty years a good deal of research has been devoted to the phenomenon, for it can be encountered in animals ranging from Man to cockroach. It has been called 'the still reaction', 'death feigning', 'sham-death reflex', 'inhibitory experimental neurosis' and 'animal hypnosis'. There are three contributory elements in the imposed situation. Overwhelming or terrifying stimulation, restraint of freedom of movement, and repetition. One or two of these elements alone will often suffice.

Some Czech experiments, involving rabbits, carried out by a

Dr Svorad, may serve as examples. The animal was held immobile and then rapidly spun round about its long axis ten
times, ending up on its back. While these alarming manoeuvres
were in progress and for some seconds afterwards, the animal's
muscles were tense and its EEG was that of extreme alertness. A
normal quadruped is possessed of 'righting reflexes' – it quickly
turns on to its feet if tipped up. The rabbits, after being whirled
round, did not. They remained motionless on their backs and
after some seconds their EEGs became transformed into the
pattern of sleep. A sudden flash of light, a loud noise, a further
forcible turning round of the body, or a brief electric shock, left
the animal still apparently sleeping with only a momentary
reaction in the EEG. Eventually, of course, awakening occurred,
leaving a normal animal. Investigating a variety of animals, of
varying ages, Svorad found it was the young ones in whom the
state of inertia and unresponsiveness could most easily be induced. The more worldly-wise old fellows took the alarums and
excursions within their stride.

The vital role which the mother, or mother-substitute, provides for her offspring, a role which is not so much that of a
snack-bar as a haven of security, and without which normal
emotional development in infancy is impossible, has been sinking
into medical minds and the public conscience in recent years. In
no small measure its impact upon medical minds has resulted
from animal experiments. Young lambs or monkeys, fed and
exercised in hygienic quarters, but lacking maternal care, neither
thrive as youngsters, nor grow into normal adults. At Cornell
University, Dr Howard Liddell has shown the necessity for
lambs to be with their mothers from the earliest hours after
birth. In the presence of the mother the world holds no terrors
for the lamb. Twin lambs were separated and one put into a
room with its mother, the other into a room alone. At regular
intervals the lights in the rooms were dimmed and, through
cables attached to a leg of each lamb, a small electric shock
was given. The lamb with his mother would jump a little, run
to her for a moment, then carry on unconcernedly. The solitary
lamb, lacking a haven of security, passed from the hostile world
into a state of animal hypnosis. It lay inert in a corner. The

shocks were then stopped but it remained asleep for half an hour, not waking if deliberately jabbed, and retaining unnatural postures thrust upon it. The mouldability is referred to as 'catalepsy'.

It could be supposed that the lamb with his mother was less afraid, and that the young animals tested by Svorad were more easily terrified than their elders. Familiarity might breed contempt. Some American experimenters tested this with hens, seizing them, and thrusting them into abnormal postures for half a minute. The hens lay inert in the odd postures as expected. Day after day the procedure was carried out on the same hens. The length of time the hen would remain inert was recorded each time. Gradually it grew less and less. As if learning that there was nothing to be afraid of, the hens soon took the procedure calmly, and eventually would respond simply by getting up and walking off instead of lying inert.

The state of animal hypnosis can be induced in monkeys. One team of workers who had been trying to decipher what were the functions of different parts of the monkey brain, and who had made localized areas of damage to various parts of the brain, found an area, which, if damaged, left the monkeys as if in a state of persistent panic. Any violent new stimulus readily provoked the state of animal hypnosis. But what really made it appear almost at the drop of a pin was simultaneous blindfolding of the same animals. Perhaps lack of reassurance through seeing the outside world was important. An equally vivid demonstration was provided by some American experiments with cats which could neither smell, nor see, nor hear. Any unusual stimulus, even if only mildly unpleasant, such as a quick tweak of the tail or a tap on the nose, would make the cat fall, quite literally, asleep. The cat was then very difficult to awaken – not surprising really, because if something like pinching would positively make the cat sleep, one would be at a loss to think how best to awaken him.

When an animal is provoked into this state of sleep its heart slows as in naturally occurring sleep. In the U.S.A., Dr Curt Richter took matters a step further. He found that, in a situation in which rats could be provoked into animal hypnosis, if he used wild rats, and if their whiskers had first been cut off, their hearts not merely slowed down, they stopped. The rats died. Domesticated rats did not die. They were accustomed to being handled by humans in a way wild rats could not be. Like the blindfolded monkeys, or the cats which could not see, hear or smell, if the rats lacked the contact with reality normally provided by their whiskers, they went unconscious all the more readily, even into permanent unconsciousness.

Dr Richter conducted these experiments in an attempt to understand the mechanism of human death as a result of overwhelming fear, following inquiries by a physiologist famous for his study of the bodily reactions to fear, the late Dr W. B. Cannon. Well-authenticated deaths following quickly upon intense grief or terror can be found among sophisticated societies as well as among many primitive peoples, such as the Australian aborigines. It is among primitive peoples, however, that it seems most common. Among, as Cannon wrote, 'human beings so primitive, so superstitious, so ignorant that they are bewildered strangers in a hostile world'. How reminiscent of whiskerless wild rats!

Human animals too can be provoked into or towards 'animal hypnosis' or sleep. There are instances recorded where dogs and cats have been trained to carry out certain actions for food rewards, but not to carry out certain others. To teach them positively not to do the latter, little electric shocks have been used. If, in these training programmes, the electric shocks have been made too strong or given too frequently, the animals have responded by falling asleep. Humans do the same. Before describing this perhaps a diversion is justified.

How different research workers first came to take up their individual special interests could fill many a story book. I became affianced to sleep by accident. Because electric shocks made a man sleep. Reading an unexciting article in a scientific journal, I happened to notice the next one. It was about people with 'number forms'. People who, if they think of, say, the numbers 1 to 20, always 'place' them in certain relative special positions. Could there be many such people? I asked around people I met. Sure enough there were such people. Some of them were vivid visualizers. They could picture a thing, stare at it for half a minute, look away and see its 'after-image' – as you will see an after-image if you stare at an electric light and then look away. One man said his after-images kept rapidly fluctuating in size. It turned out that they did so at the rate of his heart beat. Then I discovered that, many years before, comparable observations had been made. Awareness or consciousness of something that was the mind's own creation was fluctuating with the pulse. Why? Wading knee-deep into the books about consciousness, the only explanation seemed to be the carotid sinus (see p. 35). Every blood-pressure rise, with each pulse, sends a shower of nerve impulses up to the brain – a source of momentary damping of consciousness. At the rate of the pulse. Plausible, anyway. But now I was immersed in the new writings about the brain-stem regulation of consciousness, about what excited or damped the reticular formation. Experiments by anatomists with chopped-up cats. I was a psychologist. Worry kept people awake, not just noise. The cortex must stimulate the reticular formation. How to show this? Do an experiment. Use humans. Use electric shocks. . . .

The idea was to require the cerebral cortex to display discrimination in sleep by conditioning arousal to follow a certain noise. Three musical tones, each different in pitch . . . purp, poop and peep . . . were played singly and at irregular intervals. The high and the low tones, peep and purp, were never followed by electric shock. The shocks only followed the middle tone. It was when a poop was heard that the volunteer learned to expect a shock. Perhaps, if then purps and peeps sounded in his sleep he would be less disturbed by them than by poops. Actually that was eventually the case, but the important lesson for me, as is so often the case in research, came not from the original purpose of the experiment. It came in a training session. While the subject was supposed to be learning, to the point of its being automatic, that it was only the poops which were danger signals, he went to sleep. And the electric shocks only momentarily disturbed his EEG sleep rhythms.

More volunteers were persuaded to help. They went to sleep too if given electric shocks, especially if the shocks were rhythmically monotonous. 'It would never happen if they did not have their eyes shut,' my friends said. 'They must just get used to the shocks, and drop off through boredom.' The critics just never tried those shocks. There was only one way to find the answer to them. To do an experiment. An assistant and I tried first one and then another method of fixing open my eyes for an hour or so. Using glue and adhesive plaster a successful technique was eventually worked out. Volunteers (paid) were forthcoming, as is always the case (it is not just the money; there are always people about who have a zest for hazards).

Some complex gadgetry made it possible to give momentary electric shocks at a steady rhythm which was synchronized with the rhythm of four flashing lights placed just in front of the eyes, and for both to be synchronized with the rhythm of some very loud jazz music issuing from a tape-recorder. The eyes were glued open, the apparatus tested ('Those lights are so brilliant, I can't possibly stand them' – 'Oh, don't worry, you'll get used to them.' Too proud to grumble about the shocks.) Then everything switched on. It turned out to be just about the quickest way I know of getting normal, healthy humans to sleep (see p. 134). They slept, with eyes open, within a few minutes. The EEG showed its usual changes, the heart slowed, the pupils of the eyes became very small (one of the classic signs of sleep but one not usually accessible to the observer). Although the volunteers were attached to the apparatus, it was only by flimsy wires. They were harnessed, but the restraint was not physical. They were harnessed by social obligations.

How shall we interpret this sleep state found throughout the animal kingdom, which results from overwhelming or fear-provoking stimuli, coupled with physical or psychological restraints which prevent escape, with or without an element of repetition? There have been explanations in terms of purpose. The sham-death reflex may allow the hunted to escape the notice of the hunter. If unconsciousness supervenes in the face of extreme threat it may provide release from awareness of a terrible fate. The psycho-analytically oriented see it as a form of narcissistic withdrawal from unpleasant reality. Pavlov, the great Russian experimenter, who invented numerous theoretical concepts to fit his observations, concepts which are mostly not compatible with contemporary knowledge of the nervous system, also regarded animal hypnosis as protecting the brain against too violent excitement. Protect it may, but we really do not know just how it is that, instead of excitement, there may be a damping effect so extreme that apparent sleep may supervene. Some baby boys, unable to defend their property, get circumcised without anaesthetic and for a couple of days following this near-disaster they actually sleep more than usual.

The lowering of cortical vigilance may not manifest itself in so extreme a form as frank sleep, but simply by inertia and unresponsiveness. Parts of the U.S.A. are liable to tornadoes of great fury, which are terrifying for those whose homes dissolve around them. A number of studies of the immediate psychological state of survivors, and similar studies after earthquakes elsewhere in the world, have revealed what Dr M. Wolfenstein calls a 'disaster syndrome'. The affected survivors show 'absence of emotion, lack of response to present stimuli, inhibition of outward activity, docility and undemandingness'. Apart from the lack of responsiveness and inactivity, the docility is reminiscent of the compliant maintenance of some imposed posture by animals. Some years ago the Italian liner *Andrea Doria* was in a collision in the Atlantic. Two psychiatrists were able to observe the immediate survivors and remarked again how the survivors acted as if under a sedative, how they were inert and compliant.

A Dutch psychiatrist, a Jewess, has written of her four years in the Nazi concentration camp at Auschwitz. The guards always organized an unspeakable reception for new batches of prisoners, designed to overwhelm them by brutality and degradation. Those for whom the type of treatment received came as a surprise underwent 'an acute fright reaction' which was 'a state of stupor', having none of the bodily symptoms which are usually associated with fear. Hersey's book *Hiroshima* tells how, for Father Kleinsorge, the German Jesuit priest,

the silence in the grove by the river, where hundreds of gruesomely wounded suffered together, was one of the most dreadful and awesome phenomena of his whole experience. The hurt ones were quiet; no one wept, much less screamed in pain; no one complained; none of the many who died did so noisily; not even the children cried; very few people even spoke.

Helpless in the face of an overwhelming situation the reaction again was one of quiet inertia and unresponsiveness.

The reaction of inertia in face of an overwhelming situation sometimes reveals the full picture of sleep. The most characteristic single feature, however, is diminution of postural and other bodily reflexes. In animal studies, periods of animal hypnosis sometimes include a time when the EEG briefly becomes again like one of wakefulness and the pupils are dilated, yet the immobility and loss of reflexes continue. It is as if the imposed sleep were interrupted by spells during which the brain could consciously reassess the situation without completely waking up the body and losing the advantages of immobility. The state differs from another human condition which at first may appear to possess superficial resemblances but in which the person is awake and efficient, and yet is also suggestible and shows compliance with another person's behests whether communicated by verbal, visual or other symbols as interpreted by the *hypnotized* person.

Human Hypnotism

These days we have all gone very 'psychological', very understanding of human motives and relationships. Television advertisers are very understanding and imply that if a young man uses their under-arm deodorant, wears their jeans, or proffers the right box of chocolates, those delicious young women will assuredly render up their hearts. They do not, in our society, offer to sell magic potions that he should burn beneath a full moon or distil into his beloved's eyes. If a young man and a middle-aged woman marry there may be malicious comment but she will not today be accused of bewitching him with the aid of the Powers of Darkness. If a demagogue induces young men to follow his banner and obey his commands we may say, colloquially, that they have come under his spell, but we use the word 'spell' only as a figure of speech. Three hundred years ago things were different. Belief in unseen forces, in magic potions and spells, in witchcraft and malign powers, was still commonplace. If the influence of one person upon another were not clearly of God, then it must be attributable to some other supernatural power.

In the year 1679, in England, a man called Maxwell published a short treatise on magnetic medicine, attributing cures effected by this, and other unusual varieties of medical practice, to the accumulation of a subtle fluid in the body of the patient. This subtle fluid was diffused through all things in nature. A fortunate few among men had an inborn power of controlling its distribution. They could cure all manner of diseases. By adding to their own proper quantum of fluid, they would enable themselves to live for ever, were not the influence of the stars adverse.

In the year 1722 a woman was burned at the stake within the present boundaries of the city of Edinburgh. She burned as a witch. Only twelve years later was born, in a little Austrian village, a man called Franz Anton Mesmer, a man who also was one day to be accused of exerting powers through Satan. Intended originally for the priesthood, he turned to study first law, then medicine at the University of Vienna, and in 1766 received his diploma having publicly read a dissertation entitled, *Disputatio de Planetarum Influxu in Corpus Humanum* ('Concerning the influence of the planets on the human body'). Like Maxwell, Mesmer believed that a subtle fluid pervaded nature, and that he was enabled to influence its distribution. It was invisible, and so he likened it to gravitation and to magnetic force. Even today there are folk in our society who believe that the stars or the planets may modify the course of their lives.

Mesmer won freedom from material worries, and a lucrative foothold within the best Viennese social circles, when he married a rich and nobly-born widow, appropriately surnamed von Posch. But, alas, he proved unpopular with his medical colleagues in Vienna. He protested that the subtle fluid had magnetic properties, that living bodies were of two classes, one susceptible to this magnetism and one not. It was, he said, an animal form of magnetism, not requiring iron magnets.

As a sequel to the local opposition he moved, in 1778, to

Paris, where his clinic became a centre for ladies and gentlemen of fashion. His followers established the Society of Harmony. His clinic comprised essentially an exotically draped room wherein stood the famous 'baquet', a large vat filled with water and iron filings and from which projected iron bars that his patients grasped. Mesmer, armed with an iron wand, officiated in splendid robes, to the strains of music. He would gaze at the patient, pass his hands over the body and touch the afflicted part with the iron wand. The magnetic fluid being then redistributed, the patient had a 'crisis' (what we should today call an hysterical seizure) and arose, cured.

A lot of mumbo-jumbo? Yes, but effective because it was impressive. What Mesmer relied upon is still the most important factor in medical treatment. He relied upon the trust of the patient in the omnipotence of the doctor. He treated a variety of psychoneurotic disorders, certainly cases of hysterical paralysis and hysterical blindness. That is to say, he treated people who, for emotional reasons, do not use their limbs or eyes, because to do so would cause them anxiety, or lose them certain advantages. Their symptoms can be removed today, as in Mesmer's clinic, by equally impressive techniques. The sources of the emotional discontents are not thereby relieved, and it is to the latter that modern psychotherapists direct their energies.

As in Vienna, so in Paris, Mesmer found enemies. Their agitations, in almost twentieth-century style, led to a Royal Commission in 1784. Among its nine members were Benjamin Franklin, then American Ambassador to France, and M. Guillotin, whose inventiveness is immortalized in the machine to which even he himself was destined one day to fall victim.* The commissioners reported that the magnetic fluid could not be noticed by their senses, and that it had no effect on them nor on patients who were submitted to it. They concluded that

having finally demonstrated by decisive experiments that imagination without magnetism produces convulsions and that magnetism

* Mr Philip Grierson, Fellow of Gonville and Caius College, Cambridge, has pointed out to me that Guillotin did not invent the guillotine and died respectably in his bed in 1814. The guillotine was in use in England at least as early as 1695 for the stealing of cattle.

without imagination produces nothing . . . of animal magnetic fluid that such fluid does not exist . . . that the violent effects seen in public treatments from the touching, result from the imagination which is set into action, and from the machine of incitement, which we must admit against our own desire is the only thing which impressed us . . . all public treatment by magnetism must in the long run be harmful.

Mesmer died in obscurity.

A member of the Society of Harmony had been the Marquis Chastenet de Puysegur. He carried on Mesmer's work. Instead of iron rods protruding from a vat, he hung ropes from a tree with equal success. Vegetable magnetism! However, he must have adopted a rather different attitude to his patients, because some of them seemed to walk about in a manner which reminded him of sleepwalking. So he called the trance state that he had induced *somnambulism*. Other French physicians found it possible to induce somnambulistic patients to be unaware of pain, to be unable to recall things they should remember, to see or hear things not really there and not to see things that really were there. They soon found that, given a little experience, practically anyone could be a 'magnetizer'.

A Scottish physician, James Braid, who practised in Manchester, in 1841 saw a demonstration given by a French magnetizer. He tried it out for himself, and satisfied himself that the phenomena he had witnessed were genuinely possible. He adopted less dramatic devices for inducing these trance phenomena. He had his patients stare fixedly at a small bright object while he made verbal suggestions to them – a method still much used. He rejected the name somnambulism, with its Latin root, and, turning to Greek, chose to call the trance *hypnosis*.

Although there is reason to suppose that the genuine sleepwalker's cerebral cortex is functioning at a level of vigilance lower than drowsiness, the essence of his disorder is almost certainly disorientation while preoccupied. He is out of touch. The human hypnotic trance has a name that grew out of a resemblance to sleepwalking. The human hypnotic trance is not a state of sleep. Nor, let it be emphasized, is it a state of unconsciousness.

What is the human hypnotic trance? It is not possible to

categorize it in a manner that would be universally acceptable. It remains a very definite puzzle. It is certainly a state of inertia, but only in respect of spontaneous actions. In response to the hypnotist's commands, vigorous activity may ensue without disrupting the trance, or destroying the rapport. It is this rapport that is so characteristic. The hypnotized individual's own initiative is subservient to that of the hypnotist. Alternatives to that which the hypnotist suggests simply do not seem to arise. If you ask your friend to go and shut the door he may quietly do so, or he may comment that, since he sees no reason for you to be so idle, you might as well go and do it yourself. The hypnotized person just gets on and does it.

Under what circumstances do people carry out without question that which another has proposed? When the proposer possesses high prestige. When he has in the past proved to be right, especially if in the face of incredulity or opposition. Thus we find that the more impressive a person, or the ceremony which surrounds him, or the greater the prestige which his position carries, the more easily can he hypnotize others. The most difficult people to hypnotize are members of one's own family (other than children). They know you so well. They just chuckle at you. It is also a fact that while more or less anyone can be a hypnotist (though just as with tennis which anyone can play, some will be better than others) some people just are good hypnotic subjects and others are poor. It is not a matter of intellect or 'will power', nor, in any very clear way, of personality. Some people just are good subjects. With them, experiments in hypnotism are interesting and rewarding. With the run-of-the-mill subject, hypnotism is simply dull. One keeps on saying the same old things over and over again.

How is a person hypnotized? Words are the principal tools. Glaring eyes and mysterious passes are irrelevant except to impress the simple-minded. First there has to be an opening gambit, then a process during which the interpersonal relationship, the rapport between hypnotist and subject, is cemented and during which the hypnotist builds up his prestige. He progresses in little forward steps, always seeking to avoid failure, for failure will put him back several steps.

Of opening gambits there are many. Something to prevent the subject's mind being distracted from what the hypnotist is saying, to fix his attention on something of no intrinsic interest, so that he will unwittingly attend to the words being spoken to him. Staring at a bright light, having been previously told in a confident manner that his eyes will grow tired under such circumstances, staring while repeated suggestions are made about his eyes beginning to grow a little tired, how they will soon grow much more tired, how he now begins to feel the eyelids sagging, how he will soon feel them closing, how they will close, how he feels them growing heavier and heavier. And so on till the eyes close. Then comes the test. The idea having already been introduced that the eyelids will feel heavy and be difficult to open, further suggestions along these lines are made: 'And when in a little while you attempt to open your eyes, the more you try to open them the more you will feel them close tightly together, the more tightly they will close, the more firmly will the eyelids press together. You cannot open your closed eyes! The more you try, the more they go the other way! You will try, but you will be surprised to find that you cannot open your eyes You cannot open your eyes! You can try, but you cannot open your eyes!' A few twitches of the eyebrows, but the eyelids remain closed. The first hurdle is surmounted. The first prestige build-up accomplished.

Then one progresses to the next prestige-builder. 'Please hold up your right arm. That's right, quite straight. Your arm is a strong arm and all the muscles in it are strong As you think about it, you begin to feel all the muscles in your arm grow tense, tense and strong, strong and rigid. All the muscles in your arm are becoming tense and rigid, tense and rigid from shoulder to fingers, tense and rigid like an iron bar, an iron bar, straight and stiff like an iron bar, an iron bar from shoulder to fingertips, an iron bar with no joint in the middle, an iron bar that will not bend. Your arm is like an iron bar, stiff and straight from shoulder to fingertips, like an iron bar, and, like an iron bar it will not bend in the middle. Stiff and straight and rigid from shoulder to fingertips. And the more you try to bend it, the stiffer and straighter it becomes. It will not bend at the elbow,

you can try, but the stiffer and the straighter it becomes. . . .'
And so on.

And he cannot bend his arm. It is rigid and tense. The tendons at his wrist stand out like cords, sweat may pour from his brow, his body may tremble with his efforts. But he cannot bend that arm. He is engaging in vigorous muscular activity. He is not asleep.

Next the hypnotist may induce analgesia, or loss of the power to feel pain, in, perhaps, one hand. Again he does this by first implanting the idea, then working up to it as an established fact. Then he gets the subject to pinch himself or herself with the finger nails. 'Can you feel any pain? You can speak! Can you feel any pain?' 'No, no pain,' comes the reply.

The hypnotist with an eye to economy of time will then prepare the way for a quick trance induction on future occasions. 'Whenever in future you sit in a chair and look at me and I clap my hands, you will immediately go back into the state in which you are now.' This is repeated with variations and preparations are made for post-hypnotic amnesia. The subject must not remember, after the trance, that he had received the instruction about sitting in a chair and going off again at a clap. 'The memory of what I have just been saying to you is going to become confused in your mind, confused and lost in your mind, but everything will be as I have said. The memory of it is leaving you, going, going, gone. And when in a little while I have counted up to seven you will open your eyes and feel quite normal, bright and alert with a sense of well-being.' And so on.

The hypnotist can then quickly take his subject in and out of a trance many times over. The subject becomes thus a trained subject. If lucky, the hypnotist will find his subject can be induced to remain in a trance while the eyes are open. 'In a little while you will open your eyes and see on the floor in front of you a coil of rope. You will see me pick up one end of the rope and throw it upwards. The rope will remain upright of its own accord. Suddenly you will see a little Indian man, wearing a turban, walk in from your left. He will go to the rope, and climb up it. Up, up he will climb, then, suddenly, as he reaches the top, he will disappear. Then you will clap your hands and roar with laughter. You will laugh and laugh as you have never laughed before.' And so on. And the subject duly witnesses the Indian rope trick and writhes around convulsed with laughter. He has had a vision, but as you see him laughing till it looks as if his ribs must crack, there can be no doubt in your mind that this man is awake. He is hypnotized but he is not asleep.

The reader may have noticed that throughout the foregoing illustration of the techniques of the hypnotist no commands or suggestion about 'going to sleep' were used. Many hypnotists do use suggestions of sleep, or at least of relaxation, but they are inessential. Indeed, if one tries to hypnotize critically-minded persons, who are sitting up on hard chairs in a noisy room, and keeps telling them to 'Go to sleep', they are likely to tell you later that they felt irritated by the absurdity of what you were saying.

Many studies have been made of the bodily function of persons in the hypnotic trance. Breathing, heart-rate, blood-flow to the brain, muscle reflexes – all are like those of any other wakeful person and are not like those of a sleeping person. Most revealing is the electroencephalogram. Once again the EEG of the hypnotic trance is characteristic of wakefulness and not of sleep, in contrast to the state of 'animal hypnosis' described previously.

It is of course possible to send a hypnotized person to sleep, just as it is to send them into paroxysms of mirth. If he is lying immobile upon a comfortable couch while someone quietly, repetitively and endlessly drones on about relaxing and going to sleep, the drowsiness (which can be detected with the EEG) may follow and may lead ultimately to true sleep. If the latter happens, 'contact' or 'rapport' between hypnotist and subject becomes lost.

There remains a lot to be discovered about hypnotism. It is especially useful as a tool for controlling bodily functions and reducing the number of extraneous interferences during psychological experiments. But it is not a state of sleep.

7. Insomnia and Drugs that Affect Sleep

Lying awake. Tossing and turning. Mind dwelling on the same eternal problem. First one solution. Then another. Ferment. Back again to the impossibility, the insolubility. Returning, diverging. Fears and possibilities. Endless circling. It happens to everyone at times in life. They are tired, they want to sleep, but oblivion will not come.

Although there are certain quite specific mental illnesses which are accompanied by relative sleeplessness, the great majority of people who complain of either occasional or frequent difficulty in sleeping are not sufferers from mental illness. The lives they lead are simply fraught with more problems than those of others, largely because their own temperaments are such that they see more problems in life, more easily worry, have greater ambition, more responsibilities or a more easily aroused sense of guilt. It's a matter of individual temperament or personality. It is also a question of age.

In New York City a study was made of the sleep of three groups of men. Each was given a questionnaire to answer. Do you have trouble in going to sleep? Are you easily awakened? Do you have a lot of disturbing dreams? Do you drink coffee in the evening? Do you take a drug at night to promote sleep? And so on. One group of 108 men was drawn randomly from patients attending a psychiatric out-patient department at a hospital. Another, from patients attending the same hospital for 'medical' reasons such as heart, chest, or digestive troubles. A third group was made up of military personnel of as wide an age-range as possible. Obviously coughs and aches and pains can disturb sleep, but not nearly as much as worries do. Only one in five of the 'medical' patients said they had trouble with their sleep, whereas two-thirds of the psychiatric out-patients said they had sleep difficulties. The latter group attached more importance to sleeping. As expected, the healthy military personnel had few complaints about their sleep. Interestingly enough, unmarried patients, who perhaps had fewer responsibilities, were much less prone to complain about poor sleep than were married ones. Cutting across all the other divisions between those questioned was the influence of the age of the individual; older people especially complained of trouble with their sleep.

The factor of age was brought out more clearly, together with a wealth of other information, in a study carried out in Scotland by Drs McGhie and Russell. They set out to survey the ideas that average persons held about their sleep, and decided to use the questionnaire method. A list of questions was presented to each individual, together with a number of possible answers to each. The informant was required to underline the answer which seemed most appropriate to himself. He was asked when he usually retired to bed, when he usually fell asleep, when he normally awoke and at what hour he generally got up. Did he consider himself a light, moderate or deep sleeper? Was his sleep frequently broken by nocturnal awakenings? Did he feel tired in the morning? And so on.

They succeeded in collecting no less than 2,446 completed questionnaires, or about eighty per cent of the persons approached through old people's clubs, Territorial Army Units, community centres and Further Education authorities in Glasgow and Dundee. Obviously the people who completed the questionnaires were not strictly a random cross-section of the population of Glasgow and Dundee, but there seemed no special reason to suppose that the sort of person who joins a club or the Territorial Army would be likely to have peculiar sleep. The proportions of the 2,446 in the different age-ranges between fifteen and sixty-five years were closely comparable with those in the general population, as determined by the 1961 census, and the different social classes (as judged by the Registrar General's Classification of Occupations) were represented in the survey group in almost exactly the same proportions as in Scotland as a whole.

The most striking finding of this survey was the change of described sleep as age advanced. The older the informant, the more likely he or she was to report poor sleep. Seven per cent of the forty-year-olds said they generally got less than five hours sleep, but twenty-two per cent of the seventy-year-olds. As age increased a steadily rising number claimed to awaken early (before 5 a.m.) and to have wakened frequently during the night. Only five per cent of the twenty-year-olds, but nearer thirty-five per cent of the seventy-year-olds thought they kept on waking up during the night. Women more often complained of sleep difficulties than men, especially of difficulty in falling asleep. Nearly a third of sixty-five-year-old women claimed they took over ninety minutes to fall asleep, but scarcely any men found such difficulty.

If old people really do sleep less, is this because they need less? Support for this idea came from the same survey, for, whereas most complaints got more frequent with age, a complaint of morning tiredness got steadily less frequent as age advanced. But even if the elderly actually do not need so much sleep, they find it hard to believe. As age increased, more and more people who formed part of the survey, were regularly taking some drug in order to promote sleep. This was twice as common among the women, and at seventy-five years of age nearly forty-five per cent of women regularly took sleeping pills or draughts. A staggering number.

Some might be surprised by the large numbers of people dissatisfied with their sleep, and wonder if, perhaps, after all, there is something peculiar about Glasgow and Dundee citizens who belong to clubs. It is possible that those who belong to clubs actually sleep better than average. Since the Scottish survey, a Saskatchewan team has examined the relation between extroversion and introversion of personality, on the one hand, and amount of sleep on the other. They gave a paper and pencil test, the Maudsley Personality Inventory, to 228 patients as they entered hospital. This test gave a score of degree of extroversion or introversion. The patients were watched all through each night for several nights by nurses, who did not know about the results of the paper and pencil test, and a score was kept of the amount of the night each patient was thought to be asleep. Finally, the twenty-three most extreme introverts were compared with the twenty-three most extreme extroverts. The introverts slept on average under four and a half hours, the extroverts over six and a half hours. The likelihood of such a difference arising by chance from their data was calculated and found to be less than one in a thousand. Extroverts sleep better! And it is a fair assumption that extroverts are more likely to join clubs and the Territorial Army. So the guid folk of Glasgow and Dundee who answered the questionnaire may have been among the better sleepers in their localities.

On the other hand, where a questionnaire is used reliance is really being placed on the individual's own views, however accurate or inaccurate, about his sleep. Those old people who complained so much of being awake a lot in the night, were they really awake as much as they supposed? Who has not seen an elderly relative reclining before the fire, then lapsing into undignified and snoring slumber, and yet upon awakening denying having slept? We all turn over during the night, and momentarily our cerebral cortex has an EEG resembling wakefulness. Perhaps the elderly, stiff in their joints and more ready to explode into coughing, might be more liable at those times to approach more fully towards wakefulness ('I'm still awake, drat this cough'). Then, once more overtaken by sleep, they cannot make a dispassionate self-survey, 'Here I am, I'm asleep'.

In Paris, Dr Betty Schwartz has made a special study of men and women patients who claimed they could not sleep at all. In every case EEG electrodes were placed on the scalp and the sufferer climbed into bed prepared for one of those sleepless nights, having first agreed to press a signal-button whenever a buzzer sounded. In every case the EEG showed the signs of a normal night's sleep, with the usual alternation of orthodox and paradoxical sleep, and the sound of gentle snores picked up by the microphone. The buzzer was sounded many times, but no signal-button ever got pressed in reply. Occasionally the sleeper would turn over, rouse momentarily and announce triumphantly, 'There you are, you see, I'm *still* awake!' In the morning, with no memory of times when observers actually entered the room, Dr Schwartz was met with the declaration, 'I never slept a wink all night! I never closed my eyes all night!'

These patients were making estimates of time duration – duration of sleep. They were estimating it as zero. Our inner experience of elapsed time depends on how full of detail it was. When people retrospectively estimate the duration of a period of time which was, by the clock, 30 minutes, they may judge it to have lasted 38 minutes if it was full of interesting incident, but only 20 minutes if it was dull and boring. If they have received a drug like LSD (lysergic acid diethylamide) the 30 minutes will seem to have lasted a very long time, whereas if they had received a barbiturate drug it will seem to have been brief. In other words a period of mental life which is full of detail will seem long in retrospect, and a period of mental life empty of detail will seem short in retrospect. If therefore someone slept and woke and slept and woke, their periods of sleep, having been relatively empty compared with the periods of wakefulness, might well be judged to have been brief compared with what the clock would indicate them to have been.

At Edinburgh my colleague, Dr Stuart Lewis, asked volunteers who had slept all night in the laboratory to make estimates each morning of how long they had lain in bed before falling asleep, how long they had slept, and how much they had been awake. They always estimated that they had got less sleep than the EEG machine said they had, and were especially inaccurate if, having been given sleeping pills for several nights, now had the pills discontinued.

So if an otherwise healthy granny, who seems reasonably happy by day, claims never to sleep at night, we can take it with a pinch of salt. Nevertheless we should be very wrong to think that EEG waves are some ultimate criterion of good quality sleep or that there is no basis to most complaints of poor sleep.

In Chicago, Dr L. Monroe asked a large number of healthy people whether they considered themselves poor sleepers or good sleepers. He then chose to study sixteen of those who thought of themselves as very good and sixteen of those who thought of themselves as very poor sleepers. When their night sleep was studied in the laboratory it was found not merely that the 'poor' sleepers slept less and awoke more often, but that while they were asleep their sleep had less restful characteristics. While they slept their hearts did not slow down so much, nor their body temperatures fall so low. They took longer to fall asleep and got less paradoxical sleep. None of these young people was a patient receiving any treatment for poor sleep or mental ill-health, but it is especially important to note that when given pencil and paper tests of personality to complete, the poor sleepers showed up much more prone to worries and personality problems than the good sleepers.

We must bear in mind that sometimes poor sleep is a consequence of personal habits, especially intake of drinks like coffee or alcohol. My colleague, Dr Vlasta Březinová, studied the sleep of healthy people in their fifties and sixties. On some nights they had no coffee, on other nights decaffeinated coffee, and on yet other nights decaffeinated coffee with some pure caffeine secretly stirred in by the experimenter. There was no difference between the no-drink nights and the decaffeinated-drink nights, but after caffeine they slept on average two hours less and the sleep they did get was broken by awakenings nearly twice as often. Alcohol too is a common cause of poor sleep (see p. 138). So a degree of insomnia can be self-inflicted.

Many people suffer from quite severe insomnia when distressed, particularly those passing through a period of mental illness called depression or melancholia. The melancholic will keep awakening and will lie awake for hours with his mind going round and round upon unhappy themes of hopelessness and unreasoning apprehension. It is an illness which can today be easily and successfully treated, but which left to itself can persist for a year or longer before natural recovery occurs. In Edinburgh, we compared the sleep of a group of these patients with the sleep of normal men and women of the same age. The patients' all-night EEGs showed them to be awake well over twice as long during the middle of the night as the normals. Two American researchers went further, they compared another two such groups to see how easily an outside noise could cause awakening. The patients were much more easily awakened, as if within their brains was always present an easily-triggered alarm.

In Chapter 1, I described experiments which showed that a sort of alarm mechanism could be 'set' deliberately by asking someone to awaken if a certain name was audible. A minority of people are capable of setting another kind of 'alarm', an inner alarm clock, as it were, which enables them to awaken at some predetermined hour. There seems no doubt about this phenomenon, which has been objectively investigated by several research workers at different times, through studying selected people who claimed they could awaken when they chose. Japanese research workers found that such men actually woke repeatedly until the preselected hour was reached.

I have mentioned the mental illness known as depression or melancholia with its accompanying poor sleep. There was a time when it was hoped that perhaps EEG sleep research would reveal some special abnormality of brain function lying behind this mental illness, leading to a new understanding of the cause of the illness. The hopes have not been rewarded. Equally it was hoped that research into dreams and paradoxical sleep would cast new light on the mental illness of schizophrenia. Many sufferers from this illness experience false beliefs (delusions) and have false but convincing perceptions (hallucinations). We all have them while we dream. Might the schizophrenic have a much greater tendency to paradoxical sleep, so that dreams could be spilling over into his waking life? Once more research proved disappointing. There are no characteristics of the schizophrenic's sleep which set him apart from others.

On the other hand, hallucinations and delusions occur during mental disorders that we call 'organic' (because we know of definite changes in brain structure or function associated with those disorders) and, in these, sleep research really has brought a new understanding. Hallucinations and delusions occur in the course of delirium, such as *delirium tremens*. In this state, which usually lasts several days, the sufferer is restless, tremulous, fearful, sleepless, sees terrifying shapes such as snakes around him and may hear threatening voices. It is a state brought about by the sudden withdrawal of alcohol or sleeping pills from a person whose brain has become accustomed to their presence in large quantities. In the delirious period, paradoxical sleep, lasting only a matter of seconds, can be seen, by the use of the EEG machine, to intrude into wakefulness without prior orthodox sleep, and it seems likely that dream processes are here indeed being mixed up with reality.

Delirium reflects an acute, or short-term, brain impairment. Chronic, or longer-term, brain impairment is part of the inevitable process of ageing, which in some people proceeds faster or further in the brain than in others, so that we say some people are *senile* and unable to remember where they are, what day or year it is and what they were saying only a minute earlier.

The research of Dr I. Feinberg in the U.S.A. has shown that the sleeping brain reveals striking changes with age. He has studied the sleep of normal younger people, normal old people and senile old people. In conformity with what I have written earlier, the normal old people really did have less sleep and more broken sleep than young people. The senile people were worse still. The same held for other features of sleep. The aged normals got less orthodox sleep with the very largest and slowest type of EEG waves and they got less paradoxical sleep and fewer rapid eye movements. These changes were even more severe in the senile people. Dr Feinberg was able to show that these changes with age were closely correlated, step by step, with decreasing brain activity as measured by the rate at which the brain demanded oxygen at the different ages, and equally closely paralleled by declining intellectual functioning on tests of mental abilities. The younger reader may be disconcerted to learn that all these signs of oncoming senility began to make themselves first apparent from the age of thirty!

Sleep Inducers

Our grandparents lived in a society where it was thought essential to evacuate the bowels by nature, guile or force, not less than once every twenty-four hours. The older physicians of that era, and of earlier generations, had few effective weapons against ill-health. To purge the poor patient was within their powers. And how they purged! A dramatic, impressive display of physicianly skill. Today things are different. No longer is the daily laxative thought essential. The nightly sleeping pill has replaced the morning brimstone and treacle.

In the year 1953, National Health Service general practitioners in England and Wales prescribed 81,000 lb. of barbiturates. Six years later they prescribed exactly twice that figure – or 500 million sleeping pills! The rate of increase has not been so rapid since but roughly ten per cent of all general practitioner N.H.S. prescriptions are for sleeping pills and the figure continues to creep up. This does not include hospital prescribing and, naturally, no figures exist for prescriptions issued at private medical consultations.

The rise in consumption has not been confined to Britain alone. The barbiturates prescribed in Czechoslovakia doubled between 1958 and 1965. Prescriptions of sleeping pills more than doubled in Australia between 1962 and 1966, and in the U.S.A. from 1953 (when consumption was already higher than in Britain in 1962) to 1965 sales of drugs which soothe the nerves increased more than five-fold.

Is this hunger for sleeping pills a sign of some decline in moral fibre of our generation? Can we discover why people eat such vast quantities? Or offer an alternative?

One alternative for promoting sleep is on sale in the U.S.A. and some European countries, though its origins are Russian. This is the 'electro-sleep' box which delivers small, rhythmic electric shocks to special electrodes which the insomniac can fix to either side of his own head. In the previous chapter we have seen how potent rhythmic stimuli are in causing sleep, and that, if impressive (and what more impressive than electric shock to the head?), the stimuli will be of added efficacy. What remains uncertain is the regularity, over a long period of time, with which this expensive apparatus could be relied upon to induce sleep. So what! Some people just love magic boxes!

A cup of malted milk drink at bedtime has for long been a traditional avenue to restful sleep, but scientists tended to ignore it as mere folklore. Yet before the Second World War, Kleitman conducted a large and well-designed study in which he measured body movements during the night and found that, of a variety of foods, only one, a malted-milk drink, reduced restlessness, and this was true whether the drink was made with milk or water. At Edinburgh we compared the sleep of people of late middle-age after they had had a malted-milk drink with their sleep after they had taken a capsule containing, it was implied, a folk remedy for poor sleep but actually inert. It was certainly to my own surprise that sleep was very much less broken in the later night after the malted milk drink.

It is possible that this effect depends upon some special and natural chemical in the drink, or it could be just a matter of general nutrition. After all it is a basic necessity for an animal in need of food that it should hunt, and rats and cats kept short of food become very restless. One interesting study was conducted on 375 psychiatric patients in London. An observer interviewed them and assessed whether they had lately been sleeping better or worse, another assessed whether they had been gaining or losing weight, and another assessed their psychiatric state. In the final analysis it was found that recent weight gain was associated with sound sleep and recent weight loss with sleep broken especially in the later night, irrespective of depression or other mood change. Evidently an ample recent food intake is associated with sounder sleep, even if the food intake has not included malted milk, but a drink of the latter kind can ensure a credit balance and sleep less broken in the later night.

We still have not answered the question, why are so many sleeping pills eaten? They ensure a quick escape from harsh reality. The same pills, in smaller doses, are often given deliberately by day in order to relieve anxiety and restore tranquillity. Very much like alcohol. Many people who consume alcohol to excess also indulge in the pills to excess. The quick-escape action has resulted in the growth of an illicit traffic in these pills, and those who purvey them for their own profit also deal in another class of drug, called amphetamine. Amphetamine and drugs like it ('pep pills', also used as 'slimming pills' – definitely to be avoided) cause wakefulness, so that people who are drowsy

135

in the morning after too many sleeping pills feel more zippy after taking some amphetamine. But amphetamine by day means insomnia at night, so then more sleeping pills. And so on. Amphetamine will give some people a quick elevation of mood. When amphetamine is mixed with a barbiturate of the sleeping pill kind, the sleep-promoting action of one, and the insomnia-causing effects of the other, largely balance out, but the quick lift-and-escape-from-reality effect often remains, as a consequence of which mixtures of these drugs, popularly known as 'purple heart' tablets because of the shape and colour of the commonest brand, achieved notoriety some years ago because they were the object of thefts, prescription-forging and illicit intake.

When these drugs are taken, the body invariably and rapidly gets accustomed to them, or, if you like, protects itself against their effects by adjustments of nervous function which tend to restore normal sleep, mood and wakefulness. The tablets lose their effect. But the adjustments made by the body have woven the new chemicals into the bodily chemical processes, so that if the drugs are now suddenly stopped, there is a violent rebound swing away from sleep to insomnia, away from reality-escape into an irrational depression with anxiety that can be far worse than the experiences that may have originally led to the tablets being taken. So, all too often, more tablets, more tablets, in ever-increasing doses are sought. As if they could bring salvation.

Among the bodily accompaniments of this effect, one that we can very easily measure in the sleep laboratory is the variation in paradoxical sleep function. Barbiturate sleeping pills and amphetamines have some actions which are opposite in kind, but others which reinforce one another. Both taken together powerfully suppress paradoxical sleep. But the nervous systems of addicts who have taken 'purple hearts' for years have grown so accustomed to functioning in the presence of these unnatural chemicals that their sleep becomes practically normal. When, subsequently, the drugs are suddenly stopped a tremendous rebound occurs. Not only does the amount of the night spent in paradoxical sleep become about twice the normal, but it begins very soon after first falling asleep. The most striking feature of this rebound abnormality is the slowness of its disappearance. Only very gradually does sleep return to normal over a period of as much as two months.

Apart from the real addict, what of the ordinary person who, once started on a modest dose of sleeping pills, finds it so difficult to stop them? First let us consider what effects these drugs have. They decrease anxiety, they decrease restlessness in sleep, they decrease paradoxical sleep duration and decrease the accompanying dream vividness; they increase sleep duration. Some of the body's 'stress' hormones that are passed from the adrenal glands into the blood stream, the corticosteroids, which are usually present in specially large amounts in poor sleepers, are likewise reduced by these stress-relieving drugs. At Edinburgh we have done many prolonged experiments with people taking drugs of this kind. First without drugs, then taking them and eventually stopping them. We find that after a few weeks the drug effects diminish. Not because the drug has changed but because the brain has changed, so that some of its machinery is modified in such a way as to counteract the drug's effects. When we stop the drug by secretly substituting inert pills, those brain modifications that have come into being to counteract the drug remain and are left working unopposed and so we see increased anxiety, increased restlessness, increased paradoxical sleep and increased dream vividness, which, with high anxiety, results in nightmares, accompanied by high levels of corticosteroid 'stress' hormones in the blood during sleep. All these are increased above what they would have been had the drug never been taken. Sleep duration is correspondingly reduced below what it would have been had the drug never been taken. These many rebound features gradually diminish and things return to normal after the passage of a month or more.

We sometimes see much shorter-term rebounds too. Four men took inert capsules for three weeks, so giving a base-line for the amount of restlessness in the first hour of sleep, the second hour of sleep and so on. Then for five weeks their capsules contained sodium amylobarbitone and by the end of that time, sure enough, the first four hours of sleep were less restless than before the drug, but, as the night went on, sleep got more and more restless and the last three hours of sleep were much more restless than without the drug. If such restlessness can leave a memory impression it would serve to confirm in the mind of pill-takers that they were sufferers from broken sleep and encourage them to go on taking the very drug that was responsible for the restless sleep – a self-perpetuating process. There are therefore also intra-night rebounds manifest in the later hours after much of the drug has been destroyed in the body.

The same short-term, intra-night rebound occurs with alcohol. Many years ago Kleitman found that after alcohol sleep was less restless in the early night and more restless than normal in the late night. In the extreme case drunken stupor gives way to anxious, restless, morning tremor. So we could see the common complaint of insomnia on the part of the business executive as partly a result of his practice of frequent short drinks, and his tense irritability as a sign of recurrent rebound anxiety following rapid destruction in the body of the anxiety-deadening alcohol, tempting him, of course, to take another drink.

We can now understand better the violent repercussions that sudden stopping of a sleeping pill can have and why, once started, people find them difficult to stop. To stop requires a willingness to put up with broken sleep and nightmares for a couple of weeks and then even further weeks before sleep is fully normal.

The Chemistry of Sleep*

Sleeping pills do not lead to natural sleep. Not only is the all-night pattern distorted by changes in the amount of paradoxical sleep, but the actual EEG waves are changed and fast waves at about 18 cycles per second become very prominent, especially in drowsiness and paradoxical sleep. But if only we understood the natural brain chemistry of sleep, could we perhaps cure insomnia? The prospect seems to me a long way off. Nevertheless explorations of chemical substances which influence sleep are being made with especial interest in those chemicals which are known to occur in the brain.

* Some readers may find this section rather technical and prefer to skip on to the final chapter.

The great difficulty is that we know really very little about brain chemistry of any kind, quite apart from sleep, and if, for example, we give a chemical that is known to be similar to one present in the brain, we have to make a lot of assumptions in trying to interpret its effects on sleep. An example which serves to illustrate the difficulties in this field is the chemical called DOPA, which has become well known as one that benefits people suffering from Parkinson's Disease (in which the face tends to be expressionless and the limbs stiff and rhythmically tremulous).

Some research workers exercised rats to the point of exhaustion and found they then took excess orthodox sleep before paradoxical sleep. Next time the rats had similar exercise they were given an injection of DOPA and, when they slept, their paradoxical sleep was not so delayed. The Japanese experimenters were tempted to explain their observations by supposing that paradoxical sleep depended on the manufacture or presence of noradrenaline (norepinephrine) in the brain. Noradrenaline is one of the substances known to be present in the brain and known to be important in the transmission of nerve messages outside of the brain, and noradrenaline, it is believed, can be manufactured in the body from a substance called dopamine, which in turn can be manufactured from DOPA.

In the experiment it had to be assumed that the DOPA was getting into the brain and there being changed into dopamine and thence to noradrenaline which brought on paradoxical sleep earlier. Unfortunately the experimenters had no 'controls'. They did not know whether, after a second experience of exercise, the rats would have been less disturbed than after the first experience and would have started paradoxical sleep after a normal delay, quite irrespective of the DOPA. It was assumed that the manufacture of dopamine in the brain would itself be without effect on sleep and that it was the further step to noradrenaline that was the effective one. In justification, there was currently a French proposal that paradoxical sleep was a result of the actual noradrenaline manufacturing process. Yet it was already known from experiments in Chicago that a drug which prevented noradrenaline manufacture or synthesis was without effect on rat paradoxical sleep, and other research workers have since found that in some animals paradoxical sleep increases if noradrenaline synthesis is prevented. Moreover, while DOPA itself may increase paradoxical sleep somewhat in some animals, in man the opposite is true.

In such experiments it is also tempting to forget the possibility that, when unnatural amounts of one substance are given, a whole lot of other brain chemicals may be thrown out of balance, and that any one chemical may not have a single action in the brain. It could act in one part of the brain to promote paradoxical sleep and in another to reduce it, just as (p. 39) barbiturates can tend both to cause sleep and cause awakening. No less plausibly, it could act on one part of the brain to affect sleep in one way at one particular time and in the opposite way at another time, depending on how the nervous tissue was set to react to it. As an example, the 24-hour rhythm might reverse the reaction – as happens with feeding, which in rats can be suppressed by increased noradrenaline in the hypothalamus during darkness, whereas during daylight feeding is enhanced by increased noradrenaline in the hypothalamus.

Another chemical substance known to be present in the brain is called serotonin or 5-hydroxytryptamine. This substance, it is believed, can be manufactured in the body tissues from 5-hydroxy-tryptophan which in turn can be made from the amino-acid, tryptophan, present in food. Some years ago we found in Edinburgh that tryptophan taken by mouth brought on paradoxical sleep early in some people, or, in people with idiopathic narcolepsy, increased the duration of the paradoxical sleep they had when they dropped off to sleep, and in Oklahoma the effects on normal men's sleep were later confirmed. It may be that the tryptophan was producing its effect just by increasing brain 5-hydroxytryptamine but the effect might have actually been due to a change in the brain tryptamine content, or a host of other things of which we were, and still are, ignorant. Incidentally, a dose of tryptophan makes dogs and men even more lewd in outlook than usual, which is interesting when we remember the sexual features of paradoxical sleep (p. 87). I've taken tryptophan myself.

In France, Jouvet, who had thought of noradrenaline synthesis as responsible for paradoxical sleep, was intrigued by some Scandinavian studies showing that brain serotonin is located especially in a string of nerve cell groups in the very middle of the brain-stem. These groups are known as the raphé nuclei. Surgical destruction of these nuclei led to several days of insomnia in cats. Jouvet also found that a drug known as PCPA (para-chlorophenylalanine) which prevents the manufacture of serotonin in the brain, had the same effect, so it was tempting to believe that sleep depended on brain serotonin. However, Dement then found that, during PCPA administration, sleep returns to normal after about ten days, even though the brain still lacks its normal serotonin. Further strong evidence against the serotonin theory now stems from the finding that PCPA either has no effect or will actually increase sleep duration in other animals, notably men and rabbits. In favour of noradrenaline, however, having a specific involvement in the control just of paradoxical sleep is Jouvet's observation that a little zone known as the *locus coeruleus* is the crucial area in the pons; it is an area in which the nerve cells contain specially large quantities of noradrenaline and, whereas these nerve cells are relatively quiescent in the cat during wakefulness and orthodox sleep, they are very active in firing off electrical impulses during paradoxical sleep.

I think the best we can say is that, after several years of study of the possible role of noradrenaline and serotonin in the control of sleep, sleep researchers have to admit that the chemistry of sleep is as complex as brain chemistry in general, and that only advances in general knowledge of brain chemical processes will permit advances in understanding of sleep chemistry.

One further point may be of interest. Noradrenaline and serotonin are both examples of *amines*. It is believed that inside nerve cells these amines can be manufactured, stored, and destroyed, and that their destruction is made possible by an enzyme called mono-amine oxidase. I have already mentioned (p. 108) that there are drugs called mono-amine oxidase inhibitors. They prevent the enzyme working. One consequence is that the amount of noradrenaline and serotonin in the brain will increase after these drugs and this has been thought to be a possible explanation of the fact that they are successful for the treatment of depressive illness or melancholia.

When these drugs succeed in relieving depression, the depression does not improve at all when the drug is first given, but only after it has been taken for a week or two.

Another remarkable feature is that these drugs are the only ones known which will completely abolish all sign of paradoxical sleep in the human for many weeks, if not indefinitely, while they are being taken. What is more, no suggestion of abolition of the signs of paradoxical sleep is seen when the drug is first given. It only happens after a delay of a week or two, at the same time as the depression begins to lift. I have rather carefully said abolition of the *signs* of paradoxical sleep because there are grounds for suspecting that under the surface, as it were, some of the essential processes of paradoxical sleep may continue.

We now realize that lots of drugs will reduce paradoxical sleep, very few will increase it, and only a small number of brain-influencing drugs will leave paradoxical sleep neither increased nor decreased. The study of drugs will help us towards an understanding of the nature of sleep but sleep will also be a tool in exploring the characteristics of drugs because, if you want to study the effect of a drug on the brain of someone who is awake, there are not many EEG features you can measure, and, more importantly, the brain is at the mercy of a ceaseless flux of ever-changing environmental influences, or waking thoughts and fears, which cloud the effect of the drug. By contrast, the sleeping brain offers a large number of EEG features for measurement, and a relative freedom from intrusions, so that the action of the drug alone can be more easily examined.

In the next chapter I shall return to some of the things drugs can teach us about sleep and how they can give us clues to the function of sleep.

8. The Function of Sleep

In the past few years we have learned a great deal about what happens during sleep. So busy have we been asking the question 'How?', that we have almost lost sight of the question, 'Why' – what is it that sleep achieves for us? To Shakespeare's Macbeth, however, sleep was 'sore labour's bath, balm of hurt minds, great nature's second course, chief nourisher in life's feast'.

Sleep he evidently saw as Nature's great restorative. It restores the body after physical labour. We 'sleep on' a problem and see it in perspective. Restoration of buildings can utilize old materials, but in the living creature this is not possible, and instead new materials have to be manufactured, or synthesized, that is to say processes of restoration are similar to those of growth and to the endless synthetic process by which living cells are maintained in good working order. People tend to think of bones, or brain cells, as static, and that once formed, they are unchanging for ever until ultimate decay. But bones and brains are alive and in them old components are endlessly replaced by new. Restoration, repair and maintenance of living tissues are, like growth, dependent on synthesis, especially of protein. And in this synthesis what role has sleep? The role of chief nourisher, in Shakespeare's words.

We now know there are two kinds of sleep and that the brain and the body function very differently in each. I shall be proposing that each has different restorative functions and that the one somehow serves especially the body and the other particularly the brain. Of course the brain is part of the body, but not only are there two kinds of sleep, there are two kinds of synthesis in living tissues. First, synthesis for growth and repair by the formation of new cells, as in the skin, where we endlessly rub off cells while new ones form below. Secondly, synthesis for renewal of existing cells – and here we may note that, in the developed brain, synthesis of new cells hardly occurs, and maintenance and repair proceed by synthesis for renewal of existing cells alone. So it is not wholly implausible to think that the brain could require a different kind of restorative sleep from many other body tissues. Before going on to these functions of sleep, and having dwelt on the concept of synthesis in cells, I should like to turn again to the subject of rebounds in sleep.

The Paradoxical Sleep Rebound

In the last chapter I wrote that after sleeping pills were stopped it took a month for paradoxical sleep to get back to normal. Actually, careful and detailed measurements indicate that the whole re-adjustment process takes nearer two months. The same rebound increase of paradoxical sleep above normal occurs after withdrawal of amphetamine. It is a very different sort of drug, but the rebound process also takes two months. These rebounds occur where the drug has been taken for a long time and in small to medium doses. The change in the brain underlying the rebound can, however, be brought about by a single, very large dose that causes the drug to persist for days at high concentrations in the tissues, and this is what happens following some suicide attempts. We have studied in Edinburgh the recovery processes after a large variety of drug overdoses and, once more, paradoxical sleep usually takes about two months to become fully stabilized again.

Patients may be unconscious after the drugs for one day, may appear fully fit in four days, but a brain recovery process continues for long after. One is reminded of a kick on the shins where temporary incapacity may be followed by a few days only of soreness, yet the bruise takes many weeks to fade. The bruise fades as tissues are slowly repaired after the injury. We may infer that in the paradoxical sleep rebound one is seeing an indication that a brain repair or healing process, after chemical injury, is going on.

Figure 8 depicts the time course of paradoxical sleep rebounds after the sort of 'dream-deprivation' experiments Dement performed (p. 103) and after drugs. The shaded area in the lower half of the figure indicates the rebound, having a time course of about two months after drugs. The same time course for return to normality is found in many other types of brain repair following all sorts of insult. Electro-convulsive treatment (which

The Two Forms of Paradoxical Sleep Rebound

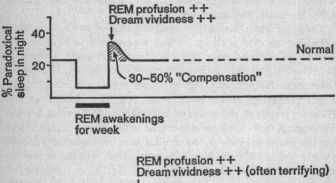

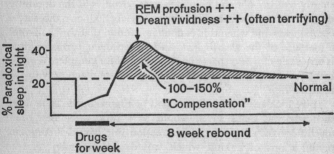

Fig 8. The upper diagram depicts selective deprivation such as Dement carried out (p. 103). The rebound is immediate and is over in a few days. The 'compensation' is small in terms of duration though there is some intensity increase.

The lower diagram depicts suppression of paradoxical sleep by a drug. The end of the drug is followed by a rebound which reaches a maximum when the last trace of the drug has left the brain. The 'compensation' exceeds the loss and there is intensity increase as well. Return to normal takes about two months, reflecting a time of repair within brain cells. Among drugs that will have this effect are sleeping pills and amphetamine.

relieves depression) causes temporarily an impairment of memory, and slow EEG waves during wakefulness, and these take about two months to disappear. Animal brains take a similar time course to recover from such things as poisonous nerve-gases. If an individual brain cell is injured indirectly through crushing of its axon (an extension along which nerve messages pass, and really part of the cell) a repair process is set in being which runs a similar time course, and in which new constituents of the nerve cell machinery are synthesized.

On p. 12 I mentioned how readjustment of brain-controlled potassium content of the urine took six weeks to adjust to a new rhythm of life and on p. 40 how brain machinery governing sleep took six to eight weeks to recover after damage. These are only some further examples of brain repair processes which begin promptly, gather momentum and then decline as full recovery is neared, the whole process taking many weeks. We can understand them if we remember that in the brain cells the working machinery is made of proteins and that the machinery is constantly wearing out and being renewed. Studies of the durability of the machinery can be made by using labelled, or radio-active, components and when this is done it is found that the 'half-life', a measure of the wearing-out and replacement turnover time, is on a scale of weeks that is just about right for complete replacement or renewal of damaged or inappropriate machinery in two months.

If we look again at the lower half of Figure 8, the time when the drug was being given would be a time when new brain machinery then leaving the production line would incorporate modifications of a kind which would, for example, tend to counteract the effect of the drug on sleep. The modifications would help to fight against the drug and so increase paradoxical sleep. After a couple of months the modification process would be almost complete. As soon as the drug stopped, the modified machinery would be left now unrestrained by drugs, to force up the amount of paradoxical sleep until sufficient machinery had rolled off the production line to bring about total replacement again. And it would require about two months.

The conclusion can be drawn that the paradoxical sleep

rebound lasts such a long time because, like other brain cell repair processes, it depends on the slowness of protein turnover through new synthesis.

The Function of Paradoxical Sleep

The conclusion in the last paragraph is one I find inescapable. However, it seems to me incomplete and insufficient and so I am impelled to take another and more speculative step.

The shaded rebound in the upper half of Figure 8 has often been called a compensation for lost paradoxical sleep. And so it may be. In duration it has never, in any of the published experiments, approached what was lost. A full compensation might, however, still be somehow achieved by an intensity increase which may be present. The shaded rebound in the lower half of Figure 8 greatly exceeds what was lost and is often coupled with an intensity increase of great magnitude. The only exceptions I know are the mono-amine oxidase inhibitor drugs, which is one reason why (p. 142) I wrote only of the *signs* of paradoxical sleep being abolished by these drugs which lead to just a small rebound.

When one sees a curve like that in the lower half of Figure 8, especially in the case of someone who has taken a drug overdose and had only a short time on the drug, one realizes that the rebound cannot be called compensation. It must be something much more, and if sleep brings restoration one has to ask why at this time, when orthodox sleep tends to be broken and of poor quality, paradoxical sleep is so enhanced. May not paradoxical sleep be essential for the brain restoration process? May it not be itself the time of most active repair by means of protein synthesis? Consistent with such an idea is the finding by workers in Massachusetts that a protein synthesis inhibitor, cycloheximide, injected into the brains of rats, has as its sequel an elevation of paradoxical sleep duration, prolonged for over a week, as if the brain was trying to overcome the effects of the cycloheximide by providing optimum conditions for synthetic processes.

There are some other facts about paradoxical sleep which

help to confirm my belief that this last supposition is a correct one. It is now known that, whereas in orthodox sleep the blood flow through the brain is at about waking levels, in paradoxical sleep the flow rises greatly above waking levels (and falls sharply in muscles). There is an accompanying rise of brain heat output. Increased blood flow and heat output are usually signs of intense activity in the living chemistry of any tissue, such as is required for increased synthesis.

There is one period of human life when not only is the total amount of sleep very great but the proportion of sleep spent in the paradoxical phase is uniquely high, twice as high as in the adult. This period is the couple of months just before birth and a few weeks after it. If one then inquires about the rate of brain cell synthetic processes one learns that they are at their highest at that very same time, and that the grey matter, or cerebral cortex, roughly doubles in thickness in the month before birth. It is possible to infer what happens before birth by studying babies born some weeks prematurely. Dr Olga Petre-Quadens of Belgium, who was among the first in these studies of premature babies, has felt forced to conclude in her writings that paradoxical sleep is specially concerned with brain growth and development. But I have already emphasized that, in living tissues, growth and renewal are comparable synthetic processes.

Dr Petre-Quadens, and also Dr Feinberg, whose studies of the senile brain I have already mentioned, have found that mentally-retarded infants and children have much less paradoxical sleep than normal infants and children and what paradoxical sleep the retarded children do get is much less intense, to judge by the fact that rapid eye movements are very sparse compared with the profuse ones of normal children. The brain of the mentally defective child is developing more slowly than normal. We believe that brain synthetic processes must be required to lay down information in memory stores and these too would be reduced in the mentally defective.

It is not only at the beginning of life that paradoxical sleep is reduced in quantity and intensity as an accompaniment of impaired brain synthesis. In senile decay the processes of brain renewal become less, and the brain literally shrivels. Senility too is accompanied by reduced time in paradoxical sleep and fewer rapid eye movements (p. 133).

The Function of Orthodox Sleep

Just as we conclude from the profusion of rapid eye movements that paradoxical sleep varies in intensity, so too we can see evidence of intensity variations in orthodox sleep. We commonly divide orthodox sleep into Stages 1, 2, 3 and 4, where Stages 3 and 4 have the slowest and largest EEG waves. They follow in sequence after Stages 1 and 2 at the beginning of the night, and it becomes progressively harder to waken someone from these successively numbered stages. In other words orthodox sleep with very large slow waves (Stages 3 and 4) seems the most intense. Stages 3 and 4 are taken in large amounts by a sleep-deprived person. They are taken mainly at the beginning of the night by all of us, namely at the time when we are most tired. When Dement and a colleague deliberately cut people short of Stages 1 and 2, as the nights went by, more time was spent in Stages 3 and 4, as if in compensation, and as if a short time spent in Stages 3 and 4 was 'worth more' than the same time in Stages 1 and 2. Men who, by nature, need to sleep very few hours take a lot of Stages 3 and 4 (p. 50).

It seems likely that orthodox sleep may be a time of especial importance for restoration in many body tissues. New York college athletes took more Stages 3 and 4 sleep on nights after strenuous afternoon physical exercise, in other words they increased their orthodox sleep intensity. Bostonian cats, after strenuous exercise, likewise had enhanced orthodox sleep. People whose thyroid glands are not passing enough thyroid hormone into the blood have very little Stages 3 and 4 orthodox sleep and are sluggish in all their activities. When given thyroid hormone, which increases the rate of energy expenditure rather like exercise does, Stages 3 and 4 increase again. People with over-active thyroid glands pouring out too much of the hormone, and so burning up their body tissues too fast, spend a great excess of their sleep in Stages 3 and 4.

All this suggested that these stages of orthodox sleep are

especially linked with general bodily restoration and so we conducted an experiment in which tissue reserves would again be burned up more than normal and we predicted that Stages 3 and 4 would increase. Ten young men first slept two nights in the laboratory to get used to it, then the next four nights to give us a base-line while they continued to eat by day, then the next four nights while they had no food at all and finally four nights while they were eating again by day. While they were fasting their Stages 3 and 4 sleep rose far above normal. Add to this the fact that at least some people who are taking a slimming drug called fenfluramine (an amphetamine derivative that helps to burn up the tissue reserves faster than normal) also get an excess of Stages 3 and 4 sleep, and it seems a fair conclusion that these sleep stages provide a specially suitable environment for body tissue restoration.

Restoration, I have said, depends on synthesis, just as does growth. It had been known for years that a particular hormone was essential for human growth, and extra amounts of this human growth hormone have been shown to increase the rate of protein synthesis in rats and in man. Then in the late 1960s researchers in Japan and the U.S.A. found that human growth hormone was released into the blood in large amounts during Stages 3 and 4 orthodox sleep. If sleep was delayed, so too was the hormone, in contrast to, for example, adrenal cortex hormones that rise late in the night whether the person has slept or not. More recently two other hormones have similarly been found to be released in large amounts during sleep, both also being hormones that help regulate tissue development, namely, prolactin and luteinizing hormone. The large secretion of these during sleep (the luteinizing hormone only during early puberty) once again does not occur if the individual stays awake. As a result of these researches it has now become common in sleep laboratories for volunteers to sleep with not only the usual silver disc electrodes on the face and scalp for picking up electrical impulses but also with a fine tube in an arm vein. At Edinburgh the tube passes through the bedroom wall so that blood can be sucked off at intervals without disturbing the sleeper at all. The blood is then spun at high speed and the clear plasma put in tubes and stored at very low temperatures to await assay of the hormone content.

Human growth hormone, like the Stages 3 and 4 sleep during which it is secreted, is higher in concentration during the night after heavy daytime exercise, after a day without food, and in patients suffering from excess thyroid production or taking slimming drugs – again suggesting that these sleep events are especially important for tissue growth or regeneration. Consistent with this is the fact that the rate of cell division, or mitosis, increases in some tissues just before or during sleep, notably in human skin and bone marrow, and in rodent skin, liver and bone marrow. It seems a sensible arrangement that, after mitotic division, along should come growth hormone to help the new cells to grow! In another Edinburgh experiment conducted mainly by Dr Ulrich Beck volunteers were awakened for an hour in the middle of the night and made to play a word-game. Allowed to sleep again they then took extra Stages 3 and 4 and secreted extra growth hormone as if to provide greater restorative action to compensate for the extra wakefulness.

Sleep for Growth and Restoration – Summary of Evidence

In this year of 1974 it may be worth summarizing evidence that now points to sleep being a time when energy is not directed to dealing with the outside world but more towards inner needs, through synthetic, or 'anabolic' processes – to an extent greater than occurs during wakefulness for at least some tissue functions.

A. Several studies do not distinguish between the phases of sleep but indicate greater brain anabolic action during sleep, for example increased incorporation of inorganic phosphate. The prolactin and luteinizing hormone favour general anabolism.

Growing animals are those that sleep the most, and a study of children with stunted growth attributed to emotional problems revealed that growth was only one third as fast at times when hospital records showed their sleep was poor.

B. Paradoxical Sleep for synthesis in the brain suggested by:
  (i) Increased brain blood flow and heat production

   (ii) Highest amounts while brain is growing

  (iii) Diminished when synthesis lags and the brain shrivels in old age

  (iv) Low amounts in mentally-retarded children

   (v) Large amounts associated with brain repair after poisoning

  (vi) Some claims of increase after extra learning

 (vii) Some evidence that it is important for synthesis of durable memory proteins.

C. Orthodox sleep, especially Stages 3+4 for general bodily synthesis suggested by:

   (i) Growth hormone, which increases the rate of synthesis of protein and RNA, is secreted in large amounts in stages 3+4

  (ii) Deliberate disturbance of the sleeper, to keep him in stage 2 and prevent stages 3+4, prevents the growth hormone secretion

  (iii) Heavy demands on tissue reserves leads to increase of stages 3+4 and of sleep growth hormone when there is need for protein conservation with (a) excess thyroid hormone (b) acute starvation (c) weight loss through slimming pills (d) heavier daytime exercise

  (iv) The longer the prior wakefulness the more of stages 3+4. A spell awake in the night leads to extra 3+4 and extra growth hormone.

The Golden Chain

I have been suggesting functions of sleep and you might reply that it has always been obvious that sleep is for synthesis or growth, because the growing infant and child seem to require so much, and that I have not really specified just what sleep does in this process. I should have to admit that this is indeed true but would reply that, if research attention can be turned to sleep as a synthetic process, a hypothesis will have been provided that can be tested through experiments. Discoveries are made in two kinds of research, research which tests specific hypotheses, and research which is truly exploratory.

The research into sleep of the last twenty years has been

accompanied by a remarkable degree of interchange among scientists who work in different disciplines. Anatomists have sat down beside psychologists at international conferences about sleep, and each has profited the other. The impetus really had two origins, the reticular formation discoveries of Moruzzi and Magoun, which they described in a publication of 1949, and the independent work shortly afterwards of Aserinsky and Kleitman studying the activity cycle of babies. They were very different sorts of study, and when I look at sleep research it seems to me that the future rests with people who are not so much specialists as generalists, biologists familiar with psychology and biochemistry. Advances in knowledge tend to flow from informal contacts between those engaged in apparently unrelated disciplines, or more especially when some individuals happen to possess a knowledge of apparently unrelated disciplines. Young research workers are, unfortunately, sometimes discouraged by their elders from pursuing interests in topics which seem outside those proper to the advancement of their career, yet a very large proportion of the major advances in fundamental research have been made by people possessing an unorthodox range of interests.

Research into the brain and behaviour is still the Cinderella of research in many countries, certainly in Britain where traditions are strong – nowhere stronger than in the medical field. Some people fear to think of the brain or of the mind; 'nerves' are still something to feel ashamed of or scoff at. They cannot face the possibility that they themselves, or a friend or relative, might one day suffer from disorder of brain and mind, whether through illness or ageing. Businessmen will subscribe funds for research into heart disease or cancer, diseases primarily of old age, but not for research into mental disorders which can cripple for a lifetime.

We already know how the death-rate from cancer and heart disease could be abruptly reduced – by less smoking and less overeating. We know so little about the brain which underlies our mental life and behaviour. This book has been about one cornerstone – sleep. Sleep, which, as Thomas Dekker wrote, 'is the golden chain that ties health and our bodies together'.

Bibliographical References

Below are listed selected references. Some are for general information and others refer specifically to items mentioned in the text of each chapter. In the latter case they appear in approximately the order in which the topics are dealt with in the chapter.

Introduction

Fisher, K. C., Dawe, A. R., Lyman, C. P., Schönbaum, E. and South, F. E. (eds.), *Mammalian Hibernation III*, Oliver & Boyd, Edinburgh, 1967.

Kleitman, N., *Sleep and Wakefulness*, University of Chicago Press, Chicago, 1963.

Oswald, I., *Sleeping and Waking*, Elsevier, Amsterdam, 1962.

Lewis, P. R. and Lobban, N. C., 'The effects of prolonged periods of life on abnormal time routines upon excretory rhythms in human subjects', *Quarterly Journal of Experimental Physiology*, 42, p. 356, 1957.

Colquhoun, W. P. (ed.), *Biological Rhythms and Human Performance*, Academic Press, New York, 1971.

Klein, K. E., Wegmann, H. M. and Hunt, B. I., 'Desynchronization of body temperature and performance circadian rhythm as a result of outgoing and homegoing transmeridian flights', *Aerospace Medicine*, 43, p. 119, 1972.

Chapter 1

Oswald, I., Berger, R. J., Jaramillo, R. A., Keddie, K. M. G., Olley, P. C. and Plunkett, G. B., 'Melancholia and barbiturates: a controlled EEG, body and eye movement study of sleep', *British Journal of Psychiatry*, 109, p. 66, 1963.

Moruzzi, G. and Magoun, H. W., 'Brain stem reticular formation and activation of the EEG', *Electroencephalography and Clinical Neurophysiology*, 1, p. 455, 1949.

Lindsley, D. B., Schreiner, L. H., Knowles, W. B. and Magoun,

H. W., 'Behavioural and EEG changes following chronic brain stem lesions in the cat', *Electroencephalography and Clinical Neurophysiology*, 2, p. 283, 1950.

Oswald, I., Taylor, A. M. and Treisman, M., 'Discriminative responses to stimulation during human sleep', *Brain*, 83, p. 440, 1960.

Rothballer, A. B., 'Studies on the adrenaline-sensitive component of the reticular activating system', *Electroencephalography and Clinical Neurophysiology*, 8, p. 603, 1956.

Arduini, A. and Arduini, M. G., 'Effect of drugs and metabolic alterations on brain stem arousal mechanisms', *Journal of Pharmacology and Experimental Therapeutics*, 110, p. 76, 1954.

Magni, F., Morruzzi, G., Rossi, G. F. and Zanchetti, A., 'EEG arousal following inactivation of the lower brain stem by selective injection of barbiturate into the vertebral circulation', *Archives Italiennes de Biologie*, 97, p. 33, 1959.

McGinty, D. J. and Sterman, M. B., 'Sleep suppression after basal forebrain lesions in the cat', *Science*, 160, p. 1253, 1968.

Chapter 2

Emmons, W. H. and Simon, C. W., 'The non-recall of material presented during sleep', *American Journal of Psychology*, 69, p. 76, 1956.

Bohlin, G., 'Monotonous stimulation, sleep onset and habituation of the orienting reaction', *Electroencephalography and Clinical Neurophysiology*, 31, p. 593, 1971.

Oswald, I., 'Falling asleep open-eyed during intense rhythmic stimulation', *British Medical Journal*, 1, p. 1450, 1960.

Chapter 3

Tune, G. S., 'Sleep and wakefulness in 509 normal human adults', *British Journal of Medical Psychology*, 42, p. 75, 1969.

Berger, R. J. and Oswald, I., 'Effects of sleep deprivation on behaviour, subsequent sleep, and dreaming', *Journal of Mental Science*, 108, p. 457, 1962.

Jones, H. S. and Oswald, I., 'Two cases of healthy insomnia', *Electroencephalography and Clinical Neurophysiology*, 24, p. 378, 1968.

Williams, H. L., Lubin, A. and Goodnow, J. J., 'Impaired performance with acute sleep loss', *Psychological Monographs*, 73, No. 14, 1959.

Zubek, J. P., 'Effects of prolonged sensory and perceptual deprivation', *British Medical Bulletin*, 20, p. 38, 1964.

Taub, J. M., Globus, G. G., Phoebus, E. and Drury, R., 'Extended sleep and performance', *Nature*, 233, p. 142, 1971.

Chapter 4

Dement, W. and Kleitman, N., 'The relation of eye movements during sleep to dream activity, an objective method for the study of dreaming', *Journal of Experimental Psychology*, 53, p. 339, 1957.

Rechtschaffen, A., Goodenough, D. R. and Shapiro, A., 'Patterns of sleep talking', *Archives of General Psychiatry*, 7, p. 418, 1962.

Foulkes, D., 'Dream reports from different stages of sleep', *Journal of Abnormal and Social Psychology*, 65, p. 14, 1962.

Oswald, I., 'Physiology of sleep accompanying dreaming', in *The Scientific Basis of Medicine Annual Reviews*, ed. J. P. Ross, Athlone Press, London, 1964.

Lester, B. K., Burch, N. R. and Dossett, R. C., 'Nocturnal EEG-GSR profiles: the influence of pre-sleep states', *Psychophysiology*, 3, p. 238, 1967.

Haider, I. and Oswald, I., 'Effects of amylobarbitone and nitrazepam on the electrodermogram and other features of sleep', *British Journal of Psychiatry*, 118, p. 519, 1971.

Dement, W. and Wolpert, E. A., 'The relation of eye movements, body motility and external stimuli to dream content', *Journal of Experimental Psychology*, 55, p. 543, 1958.

Berger, R. J. and Oswald, I., 'Eye-movements during active and passive dreams', *Science*, 137, p. 601, 1962.

Gross, J., Byrne, J. and Fisher, C., 'Eye movements during emergent stage 1 EEG in subjects with life-long blindness', *Journal of Nervous and Mental Disease*, 141, p. 365, 1965.

Molinari, S. and Foulkes, D., 'Tonic and phasic events during sleep: psychological correlates and implications', *Perceptual and Motor Skills*, 29, p. 343, 1969.

Gottschalk, L. A., Stone, W. N., Gleser, G. C. and Iacono, J. M., 'Anxiety levels in dreams: relation to changes in plasma-free fatty acids', *Science*, 153, p. 654, 1966.

Hall, C. S., 'A cognitive theory of dream symbols', *Journal of General Psychology*, 48, p. 169, 1953.

Berger, R. J., 'Experimental modification of dream content by meaningful verbal stimuli', *British Journal of Psychiatry*, 109, p. 722, 1963.

Witkin, H. A. and Lewis, H. B., 'The relation of experimentally induced presleep experiences to dreams', *Journal of the American Psychoanalytic Association*, 13, p. 819, 1965.

Baekeland, F. and Lasky, R., 'The morning recall of rapid eye movement period reports given earlier in the night', *Journal of Nervous and Mental Disease*, 147, p. 570, 1968.

Karacan, I., Goodenough, D. R., Shapiro, A. and Starker, S., 'Erection cycle during sleep in relation to dream anxiety', *Archives of General Psychiatry*, 15, p. 183, 1966.

Pai, M. N., 'Sleep-walking and sleep activities', *Journal of Mental Science*, 92, p. 756, 1946.

Kales, A., Jacobson, A., Paulson, M. J., Kales, J. D. and Walter, R. D., 'Somnambulism: psychophysiological correlates', *Archives of General Psychiatry*, 14, p. 586, 1966.

Chapter 5

Jouvet, M., 'Recherches sur les structures nerveuses et les mécanismes responsables des différentes phases du sommeil physiologique', *Archives Italiennes de Biologie*, 100, p. 125, 1962.

Frederickson, C. J. and Hobson, J. A., 'Electrical stimulation of the brain stem and subsequent sleep', *Archives Italiennes de Biologie*, 108, p. 564, 1970.

Oswald, I. and Thacore, V. R., 'Amphetamine and phenmetrazine addiction: physiological abnormalities in the abstinence syndrome', *British Medical Journal*, 2, p. 427, 1963.

Dement, W. C., 'The effect of dream deprivation', *Science*, 131, p. 1705, 1960.

Fisher, C. and Friedman, S., 'On the presence of a rhythmic, diurnal, oral instinctual drive cycle in man: a preliminary report', *Journal of the American Psychoanalytic Association*, 15, p. 317, 1967.

Oswald, I., Merrington, J. and Lewis, H., 'Cyclical "on demand" oral intake by adults', *Nature*, 225, p. 959, 1970.

Costello, C. G. and Smith, C. M., 'The relationships between personality, sleep and the effects of sedatives', *British Journal of Psychiatry*, 109, p. 568, 1963.

Schoenenberger, G. A., Cueni, L. B., Monnier, M. and Hatt, A. M., 'Humoral transmission of sleep. VII Isolation and physical–chemical characterization of the "sleep-inducing factor delta"', *Pflügers Archives für die gesamte Physiologie des Menschen und der Tiere*, 338, p. 1, 1972.

Fencl, V., Koski, G. and Pappenheiner, J. F., 'Factors in cerebrospinal fluid from goats that affect sleep and activity in rats', *Journal of Physiology*, London, 216, p. 565, 1971.

Bibliographical References

Chapter 6

Gilman, T. T., Marcuse, F. L. and Moore, A. U. 'Animal hypnosis: a study in the induction of tonic immobility in chickens', *Journal of Comparative and Physiological Psychology*, 43, p. 99, 1950.

Carli, G., 'Dissociation of electro-cortical activity and somatic reflexes during rabbit hypnosis', *Archives Italiennes de Biologie*, 107, p. 219, 1969.

Richter, C. P., 'On the phenomenon of sudden death in animals and man', *Psychosomatic Medicine*, 19, p. 191, 1967.

Emde, R. N., Harmon, R. J., Metcalf, D., Coenig, K. L. and Wagonfeld, S., 'Stress and neonatal sleep', *Psychosomatic Medicine*, 33, p. 491, 1971.

Wolfenstein, M., *Disaster. A Psychological Essay*, Routledge & Kegan Paul, London, 1957.

Chapter 7

Weiss, H. R., Kasinoff, B. H. and Bailey, M. A., 'An exploration of reported sleep disturbance', *Journal of Nervous and Mental Disease*, 134, p. 528, 1962.

McGhie, A. and Russell, S. M., 'The subjective assessment of normal sleep patterns', *Journal of Mental Science*, 108, p. 642, 1962.

Latash, L. P. and Danilin, V. P. 'Subjective estimation of the duration of time periods in night sleep', *Nature*, 236, p. 94, 1972.

Monroe, L. J., 'Psychological and physiological differences between good and poor sleepers', *Journal of Abnormal and Social Psychology*, 72, p. 255, 1967.

Zung, W. W. K. and Wilson, W. P., 'Time estimation during sleep', *Biological Psychiatry*, 3, p. 159, 1971.

Feinberg, I., Koresko, R. L. and Heller, N., 'EEG sleep patterns as a function of normal and pathological aging in man', *Journal of Psychiatric Research*, 5, p. 107, 1967.

Oswald, I., 'Drug research and human sleep', *Annual Review of Pharmacology*, 13, p. 243, 1973.

Jouvet, M., 'Biogenic amines and the states of sleep', *Science*, 163, p. 32, 1969.

Wyatt, R. J., 'The serotonin-catecholamine-dream bicycle: a clinical study', *Biological Psychiatry*, 5, p. 33, 1972.

Chernik, D. A., Ramsey, T. A., Mendels, J., 'The effect of parachlorophenylalanine on the sleep of a methadone addict', *British Journal of Psychiatry*, 122, p. 191, 1973.

Perez-Cruent, J., Tagliamonte, A., Tagliamonte, P. and Gessa, G. L.,

'Differential effect of p-chlorophenylalanine (PCPA) on sexual behavior and on sleep patterns of male rabbits', *Rivista di Farmacologia e Terapia*, 11, p. 27, 1971.

Chapter 8

Haider, I. and Oswald, I., 'Late brain recovery processes after drug overdose', *British Medical Journal*, 2, p. 318, 1970.

Goas, J. Y., Seylaz, J., Mamo, H., Macleod, P., Caron, J. P. and Houdart, R., 'Variations du débit sanguin du cortex de l'homme au cours du sommeil', *Revue Neurologique*, Paris, 120, p. 159, 1969.

Sassin, J. F., Parker, D. C., Mace, J. W., Gotlin, R. W., Johnson, L. C. and Rossman, L. G., 'Human growth hormone release: relation to slow-wave sleep and sleep-waking cycles', *Science*, 165, p. 513, 1969.

Fisher, L. B., 'The diurnal mitotic rhythm in the human epidermis', *British Journal of Dermatology*, 80, p. 75, 1968.

Sassin, J. F., Frantz, A. G., Kapen, S. and Weitzman, E. D., 'The nocturnal rise of human prolactin is dependent on sleep', *Journal of Clinical Endocrinology and Metabolism*, 37, p. 436, 1973.

Boyar, R., Funkelstein, J., Roffwarg, H., Kapen, S., Weitzman, E. and Hellman, L., 'Synchronization of augmented luteinizing hormone secretion with sleep during puberty', *New England Medical Journal*, 287, p. 582, 1972.

Wolff, G. and Money, J., 'Relationship between sleep and growth in patients with reversible somatotropin deficiency (psychosocial dwarfism)', *Psychological Medicine*, 3, p. 18, 1973.

Adamson, L., Hunter, W. M., Ogunremi, O. O., Oswald, I. and Percy-Robb, I. W., 'Growth hormone increase during sleep after daytime exercise', *Journal of Endocrinology* (in press), 1974.

Index

More about Penguins and Pelicans

Penguinews, which appears every month, contains details of all the new books issued by Penguins as they are published. From time to time it is supplemented by *Penguins in Print*, which is a complete list of all titles available. (There are some five thousand of these.)

A specimen copy of *Penguinews* will be sent to you free on request. For a year's issues (including the complete lists) please send £1 if you live in the British Isles, or elsewhere. Just write to Dept EP, Penguin Books Ltd, Harmondsworth, Middlesex, enclosing a cheque or postal order, and your name will be added to the mailing list.

In the U.S.A.: For a complete list of books available from Penguin in the United States write to Dept CS, Penguin Books Inc., 7110 Ambassador Road, Baltimore, Maryland 21207.

In Canada: For a complete list of books available from Penguin in Canada write to Penguin Books Canada Ltd, 41 Steelcase Road West, Markham, Ontario.

Dreams and Nightmares

J. A. Hadfield

Dreams have a fascination for everyone, partly because of their bizarre nature, partly because these strange imaginings come from within ourselves, and partly because of the effect they have upon our daily lives. It is not surprising that efforts at dream interpretation have been made throughout all ages, by the most primitive tribes, who regard them as premonitions, no less than in the attempts at establishing a scientific method made by Freud with his sexual wish-fulfilment theory, Jung with his archetypes from the racial subconscious, and Adler with his urge to power. In this book Dr Hadfield attempts to show that dreams have a biological role, and may be useful in the solution of the practical everyday, as well as of the deep-rooted, problems of our life. Many mathematical problems have been solved in dreams, and many scientific discoveries made by their means. We cannot, therefore, afford to ignore the significance of our dreaming, just as we cannot afford to ignore that of our intuition. This book, then, is a brief sketch of the mechanism, nature, and importance of our dream life.

Hypnosis: Fact and Fiction

F. L. Marcuse

This book attempts to offer a broad view of the field of hypnosis. It answers questions frequently asked by students and non-students alike, and to both classes of readers presents new material of interest and importance. In addition to discussing some of the general problems of hypnosis, it is also concerned with applications (clinical, medical, dental, and so on), techniques, dangers (real and imagined), theories (sleep, conditioning, etc.), and attitudes (academic, religious, medical). The book's main purpose is to separate fact from fiction in this highly controversial field.

The viewpoint of the author is not that hypnosis offers a panacea or a magical solution of the problems of psychopathology, but rather that it is a technique which is often of value and that its study can add important new data to our knowledge of human behaviour.